KETO BBQ

Real Barbecue for a Healthy Lifestyle

Myron Mixon

Written with Kelly Alexander

Abrams, New York

TABLE OF CONTENTS

KETO BBQ

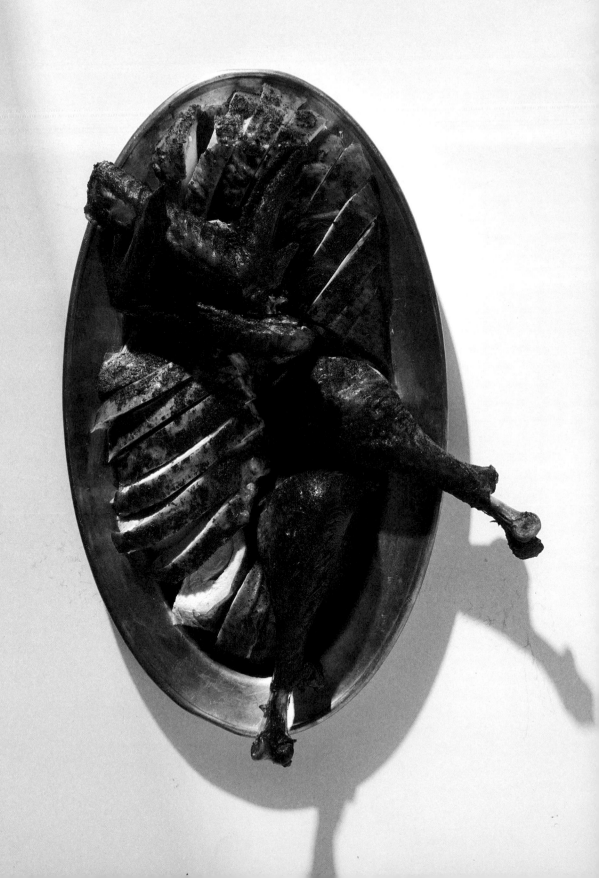

CHAPTER 8: Drinks   171

There is no eating plan on earth that I would follow if I couldn't have a cocktail or two when I felt like it.

A Note About Restaurants & Exercise   185

My tips and tricks for how to sort through any restaurant menu to stay on the diet plus an explanation of how I went from doing zero exercise to building up to a consistent and doable workout routine. If I can, you can.

The Keto BBQ Team   101

Index   194

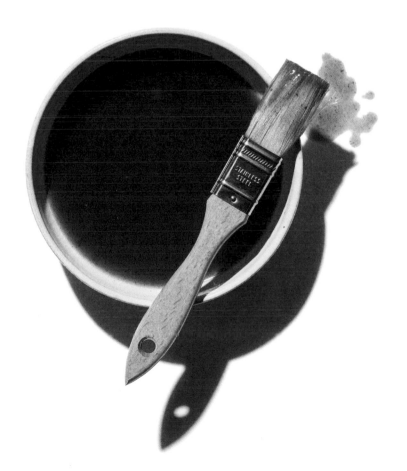

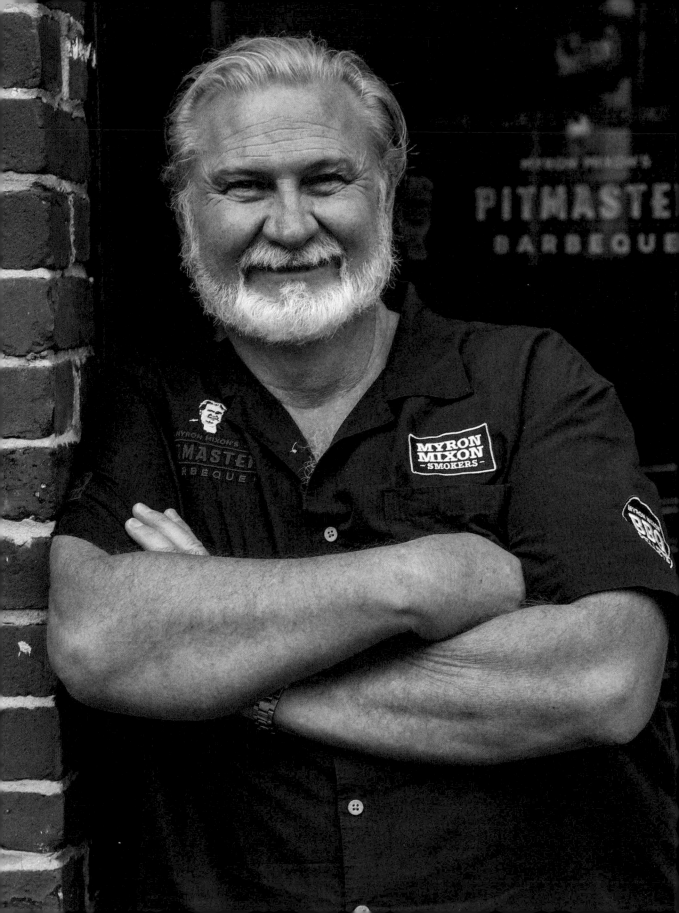

How I learned to
lose weight *and keep it off*
while eating a whole lotta BBQ

DEAR BARBECUE FANS, let's face it: For most of us, there comes a point in our lives when we need to lose weight.

Look at the numbers. According to the writer I pay to work with me on this book and the latest data from the Centers for Disease Control, whose headquarters in Atlanta are not far from my hometown of Unadilla, Georgia, 72% of adults over the age of twenty in America today are overweight, which means they weigh more than they should for their given height and have what doctors consider an elevated body mass index. The exact number of overweight people matters less than the problem itself does: If you weigh more than your bones are supposed to carry, you're in line for a whole bunch of associated health problems. Everyone knows that, even world-championship-winning barbecue pitmasters like me.

When it happens to you, you have to decide what to do about it. You can blame it on genetics, on your metabolism slowing down, or on one of a thousand other reasons you can come up with—but there's no easy way to bring down the number you see on that scale.

For me, I became overweight for the simple reason that I put too much food in my mouth. I'm talking about a lot of food, and I had gotten away with eating that way for a long time without the effects catching up to me. As a kid, my granny used to fry up all the pieces from three whole chickens just for me and my brother Tracy to enjoy. Growing up in the South, it was not unusual for young boys like us to put away three whole chickens, along with sides of rice, gravy, and biscuits.

Somehow, I was able to eat like that into my early forties without becoming excessively overweight. It probably had a lot to do with the fact that I was traveling all around the country competing at barbecue contests and working my ass off to win them. That's all I cared about back then, and the intensity that I put into it kept me fit.

Then I hit my fifties. I was still traveling all around the country and the world competing in smoking contests, but I now was also exerting a lot of energy and time supporting my growing barbecue business. This meant promoting my smokers and other products, taping television shows, opening restaurants, and doing live smoking demos. Even though I was still on my feet a lot, I wasn't getting as much exercise as I had when I was on the competitive barbecue circuit fulltime and working outdoors all day. Plus, I was eating junk food and I was eating it at all different times of the day and night because I was on the road so much. I didn't realize it, but I was doing all of the things that people shouldn't do if they want to stay healthy. Yet, despite that I had gotten heavier and heavier, I didn't take it particularly seriously. I would go to my doctor every year for my check-up, and because my blood pressure was somehow still perfect and my cholesterol and blood sugar numbers were decent, too. I could easily justify how I was eating.

Oddly enough, what eventually got to me were not medical issues but what I call "miserable issues." I weighed myself on August 8, 2018. I am a little over six feet tall, and I weighed 339 pounds! The writer I work with looked it up and told me that I weighed a good 100 pounds more than someone my height should weigh. I didn't need her to tell me this; I felt it.

"It's hell to have a two-ton body on a one-ton chassis."

And I mean, I felt it in my bones. All that extra weight I was carrying caused me shortness of breath and I began to have a hard time moving around, let alone trying to do any exercise—even walking on a treadmill got me winded fast. My hips, knees, and feet were screaming from that extra person I was carrying around. As my good friend Jamie Gear who builds barbecue pits in Texas says, "It's hell to have a two-ton body on a one-ton chassis."

I had to do something. At first, I tried to do what most doctors tell us weight-challenged folks to do: Eat small portions of all the food groups for a balanced diet. This advice comes from the theory that it ain't what you're eating that makes you fat, but how much of it. I agree with that . . . in theory. Because I'm also a realist, I knew I loved bread and dessert, and I know what I can and cannot eat. The well-balanced, small portion diet allows you to have a little bread, a few sweets, a little bit of mashed potatoes, a little bit of blah blah blah . . . and that ain't gonna cut it with me. There was just no way that I could go from eating half a package of dinner rolls at supper to feeling satisfied with just one roll.

So, what was going to work for me? Experience told me that for a diet to succeed, it has to be two things: First, it's got to be easy to follow. Second, it's got to be sustainable for the future. If it's not those two things, a person might lose weight but eventually put it back on again. I knew that for me every time I tried one of those blah blah diets, the weight I lost came right back once I stopped paying careful attention to portions and started living again. For me, any diet that allows for consuming meat was the best choice. I'm a BBQ man. I was raised eating any and every cut of meat, fowl, or fish that can be smoked or grilled—and that includes tails, cheeks, trotters, and snouts. This attitude conveniently fit in with the fact that every diet I have ever heard of that has managed to make a lasting difference in the lives of people over time was one that was low in carbohydrates.

My beloved barbecued foods have gotten a bad rap over the years when it comes to people believing that they're not as healthy for you as other foods. That isn't strictly true. How could it be, since grilling and smoking meats is a lot better for you than frying them or covering them in butter or oil or fattening sauces? It struck me that the reason people think barbecue is unhealthy is because of the side dishes that come with the meat. The part of a barbecue meal that puts the weight on y'all is usually the potato salads, hushpuppies, and helpings of mac 'n' cheese. And let's not forget about ingredients like brown sugar and corn syrup that go into a lot of barbecue sauce recipes. Those ain't helping your belly or your butt, either.

It dawned on me then that I was going to have to go cold turkey. Yes, I realized that the easiest and best way for me to stay healthy was to up and quit the foods that cause us all to gain weight—like bread, sugar, and anything fried. To replace them, I started looking at some low-carb alternatives to see what else was out there. The problem was that I wasn't going to eat most of the damn foods that the so-called experts suggested. I'm not going to eat a pizza made out of cauliflower, know what I mean? I started thinking about the food I could eat on a low-carb diet and I quickly saw that barbecue could be my salvation! If it is done right, it could be the hero food that we've all been waiting for when we try to lose weight. I saw that yes, there was a way to have our ribs without getting any fatter than the pig they came from. Clearly, I was going to have to devise my own version of one of those diets, one that would allow me to maximize eating the smoked and grilled foods I'm known for cooking better than anyone else. So, I sat down and started planning and experimenting with the barbecue foods I like and that also fit into a low-carb diet. That's how this book was born.

I built my own diet plan around the "Keto" diet. This is a term that's been used to death. When I first heard it, I thought it sounded like something you'd hear in a game of *Mortal Kombat*. After the writer I hired did some research, I found out that the name comes from "ketosis"—the scientific word for the body's state when fat provides the majority of the body's fuel (instead of, say, carbs). The bottom line with Keto, as I'm told, is that it's a diet built around eating a lot of proteins and healthy fats (like avocados, as opposed to doughnuts), very few carbs, and no sugar. Since our bodies normally burn carbs for energy, the Keto diet changes it up. If you limit carbs and increase fat, your body converts the fat into energy and burns it off in a more efficient way. This approach sounded perfect for the full-figured man I was.

I'm sure by now you all want to know if the "BBQ Keto" diet plan I created for myself worked. Here's the big reveal, as they say on those weight-loss television shows. As I told you when I started my diet plan on August 8, 2018, I weighed 339 pounds and had a 46-inch waist. After nine months on the diet, I was down to 235 pounds, with a 36-inch waist. And I have kept it like that ever since. I have even been able to add exercising, which I couldn't physically do until I got rid of some of that weight. Now I walk, treadmill, and do weight training, too. In this book, I'm going to give you a roadmap for how I did it. My plan is one that all of you backyard pitmasters can easily follow. I know you'll be able to do it because I did.

Trust me when I tell you that the rewards are huge. One cool thing I have found is that after you get your weight off and have sustained it for a while, you can have some whole grain bread or some dessert, if you like. It comes down to you deciding if you have the kind of willpower and discipline to sample those items without going hog wild and blowing your routine. A big problem with most diets is feeling like you can't go out to eat because there won't be anything for you on the menu. My Keto diet is not about deprivation. It's about eating grilled and smoked meats and losing weight. That means that when I go to a restaurant, I can always find something to eat—and I'm gonna give you all the tips you need to both cook your own and order meals that'll be complementary to this plan.

If you think that losing weight while regularly enjoying spareribs, grilled chicken, smoked turkey, and beef brisket sounds good, then fire up the smoker and join me. These foods are just the tip of the BBQ foods Keto collection I've put together for you.

Keep smokin',
Myron

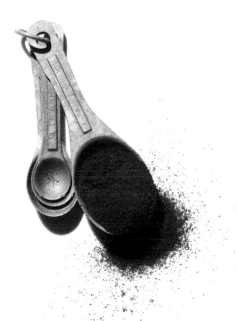

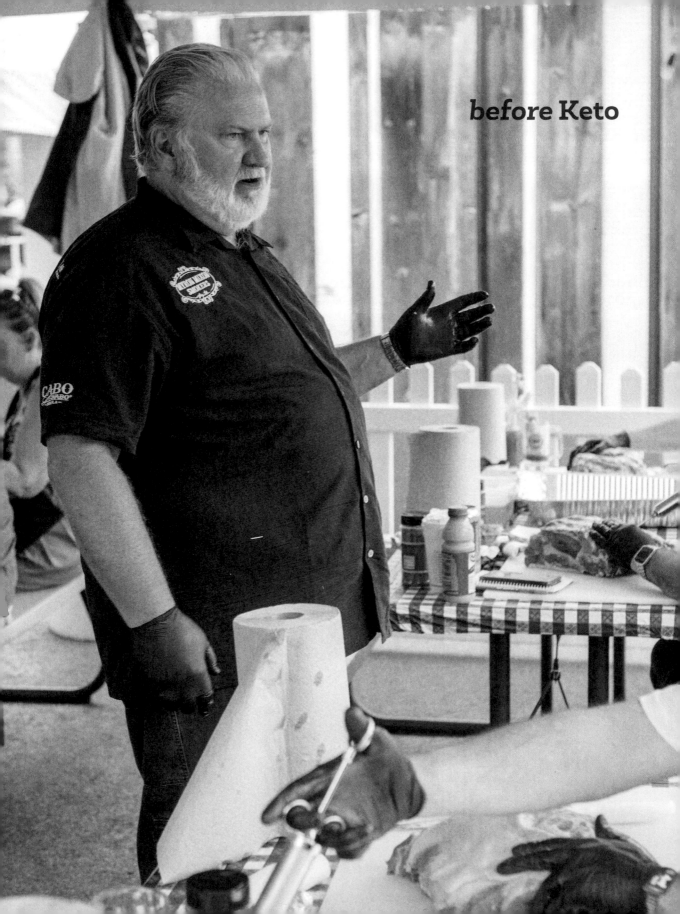

before Keto

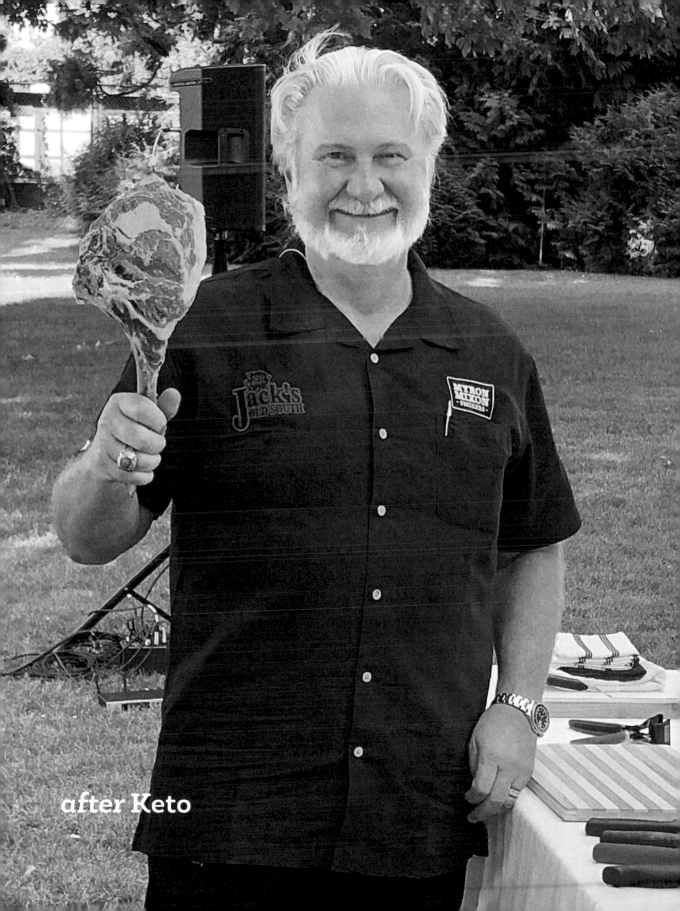

after Keto

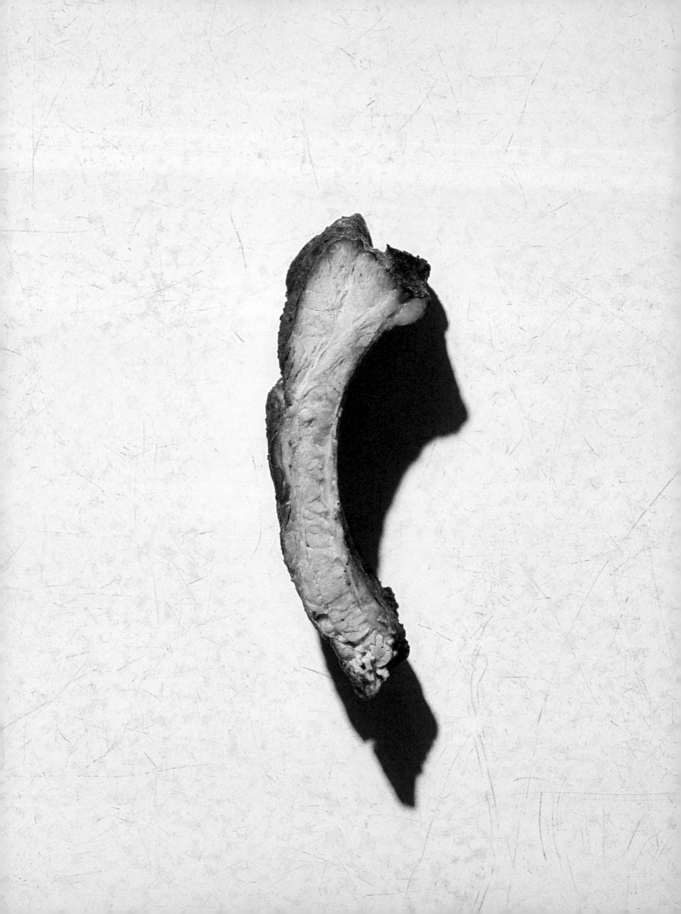

CHAPTER 1

Keto Cooking
for Pitmasters

DISCLAIMER: Folks, I am the winningest man in barbecue, a four-time world champion who has taken first place in every single barbecue cooking contest that matters in this world—state championships, regional championships, local championships, too. Kelly Alexander, the writer I pay to put down my wisdom in words that fill my books is a damn PhD. She's got her doctorate in food studies and teaches college classes. We're a good team, but neither one of us is a nutritionist or a dietician. We don't work at the Mayo Clinic or in a hospital, and we both try to stay out of places like that. So, we're not going to give you what one might call "an exhaustive review" of the Keto diet because neither one of us is qualified to explain how healthful it is without getting sued. However, we both happen to believe based on our own experiences losing weight on the Keto diet and feeling good in the process that it has a bunch of benefits. Think about it: If you eat less sugar and lose weight, wouldn't you also move better, sleep better, have better blood pressure levels, and even have better skin? You know you would.

Here are the basics to the diet as I have followed it, plus my ideas for the best ways to get yourself up and running so you can start smoking meat and enjoying being skinny, like I am now.

What the hell is Keto?

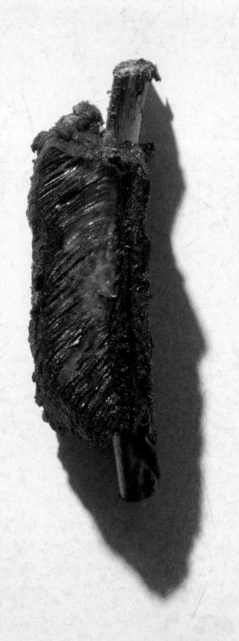

In a nutshell, the Keto diet is a super low-carbohydrate diet that includes a high level of healthy fats and a moderate level of protein. If you can wrap your mind around that, you've pretty much got the gist.

Other useful facts:

Even though it's trendy and people throw the word "Keto" around a lot, a Keto plan is not a crash diet. When I think of crash diets, I think of eating plans that restrict your calories to near-starvation levels so that you can lose weight, but the minute you return to living your life with a more sustainable level of food, you gain it all back. This is one reason I like Keto: It does not restrict calories.

Sounds great, you can eat as much as you want right? Yes, that's true, but you can't eat as much as you want of whatever you want. Keto doesn't involve counting calories, but you do have to cut out, avoid, and drastically limit certain foods. That means cutting out sugar, starches, and grains. That means limiting fruits that contain high levels of sugar. That means no more sandwiches for lunch and no more spaghetti for dinner. You think that sounds hard? I don't even want to hear it. I've had to do much harder stuff in my life, and I'm sure you have, too. Winning the world championship of barbecue four times is much more difficult. So is figuring out how to support your family after you've just gotten a divorce, your dad just died, and you've got two kids and a truck payment. I say you can do it. Put down that piece of pizza, pick up a smoked chicken leg, and keep it moving with your weight loss goals. That's what the recipes in this book are here to help you do: Satisfy cravings you may have for high-carb foods and adjust to a new way of eating that is delicious and also helps you lose weight and keep it off in a way that I know works because I'm living proof.

For the science-minded among you, from the research my writer has done, here's what we can tell you: The name "Keto" comes from the term "ketosis," a physical state in which a body uses fats, rather than the sugars from carbohydrates, to fuel itself. Getting most of your calories from fat forces your body to use different energy pathways than it is used to using. If you want to understand all of this, you need to know how your body stores energy from food. The body typically likes to get its energy from carbs, which are its go-to sources. But if you don't eat any carbs, the body burns fat instead. If your body burns fat instead of carbs and sugars, you're said to be "in ketosis." The Keto diet works by getting your body to go into ketosis—and, by not eating carbs, keeping it that way. The key is to keep your food intake at 70 to 75 percent healthy fats, 20 to 25 percent protein, and about 5 percent carbs. That's the formula you're supposed to follow, anyway, and some people do it very religiously—they buy something called a "Keto macro calculator" to help track their nutrient consumption every day. You can do that if you like—if you're the kind of person who finds numbers soothing and needs extra support. I just monitor what I eat and track my carbs by watching what I put in my mouth. That's more or less what you need to know: The Keto diet is designed to turn your body into a fat-burning machine. The rest of it, you can read up on it in the hundreds of science and nutrition textbooks out there. If you don't feel like getting a degree in nutrition, I've told you all you to need to know.

How do I get started?

What I like most about Keto—after the number of pounds I've lost doing it, of course—is that it's very easy to follow when cooking at home as well as eating out. The recipes I'm going to give you are simple and use familiar foods you probably already have in your pantry. If you follow my advice, I can show you how to turn everyday ingredients into Keto-friendly meals full of healthy fats and proteins your body will use to fuel itself. The most important step in starting is: Just start.

You're going to want to stock up on Keto-friendly foods, which I can help you with in my recipes. But you're also going to want to have stuff on hand for when those inevitable carb-cravings happen (and they will, every time you watch *The Great British Baking Show*, for example). The first thing you need to do is get rid of the low-fat, high-carb foods in your pantry. That means flour, bread, rice, and sugar. Look at it this way: If you don't have the ingredients sitting around to make your favorite cake with, you can't be tempted to make it.

Cutting excess sugar out of your life is the first step—that means brown sugar, white sugar, honey, molasses, agave, maple syrup—all that stuff you use to sweeten your food. It's not high-quality fuel for your body, and what's more I guarantee that it makes you fat! Look into your pantry and get rid of all the obvious contenders. Now get rid of anything that has the following on its nutrition label: acesulfame potassium (Ace-K, Sunette), aspartame, cane sugar, dextrose, fruit juice concentrate, glucose-fructose corn syrup, high-fructose corn syrup, maltodextrin, mixed artificial sweeteners (Equal), saccharin (Sweet'N Low), sacchar ose, sucralose (Splenda), and sucrose. Even though some of the artificial sweeteners on this list have no calories, they trick your body into thinking they're sugar and trigger cravings and thus in the end have the same effects as sugar: they make you fat.

Note About Monk Fruit Sweetener

There are so many "alternative sweeteners" out there on the market that when I first started following a Keto plan, I didn't know which one try and what the difference was. You can thank me now; I tried a whole bunch of them, so now you don't have to. The one I like best is a product made from the Chinese mountain-orchard melon called monk fruit. This sweetener is extracted from that fruit (that's why you some-times see it called "monk fruit extract") and a little goes a long way: I read that scien-tists estimate monk fruit sweetener is 150 to 250 times as sweet as sugar. That's no big deal, and means you just need a smaller amount of it in, say, your barbecue sauce recipe. One thing I especially like about monk fruit sweetener is that it's natural and fruit based. I warn you that it is not the cheapest alternative sweetener out there, but I think it's worth the extra few dollars when you don't have to worry about either added chemicals or calories. Make sure when you buy it that you don't get a version that has been mixed with other sweeteners, starches, or stabilizers—you want your monk fruit sweetener to have one ingredient in it.

KETO FOODS I ENJOY:

MEATS

Beef
(ground beef, steak, brisket, etc.)
Chicken

Duck
Goose
Lamb & Mutton

Pork
(chops, ribs, roasts, smoked shoulders, hams, loins, bacon, etc.)

Sausage
(without fillers)
Turkey
Venison

SEAFOOD & FISH

Crawfish
Crab

Fish
Lobster

Mussels
Scallops

Shrimp

DAIRY

All types of cheese
(blue cheese, cheddar, mozzarella, provolone, ricotta, etc.)
Cottage cheese
Cream cheese
Eggs

Greek yogurt and regular yogurt
(full fat varieties, and none with added sugar, so watch out for the flavored varieties and check your labels)

Heavy cream
Ranch and blue cheese salad dressing
(so long as there's no sugar added, or make your own, see my recipe on page 163)

Unsweetened almond, oat, coconut, and other milk

NUTS & SEEDS

Almonds
Brazil nuts
Hazelnuts

Macadamia nuts
Peanuts
(in moderation)

Pecans
Pine nuts
Pumpkin seeds

Sesame seeds
Walnuts

FRUITS & VEGETABLES

Asparagus
Avocados
Bell peppers
Blueberries
Blackberries
(this is my all-time favorite snack, see page 147 for how I zest them up)

Broccoli
Cabbage
Carrots
(in moderation)
Cauliflower
Celery
Coconut
Cucumbers
Green beans

Lemons
Limes
Mushrooms
Okra
Olives
Onions
Pickles
Pumpkin
Radishes

Raspberries
Salad greens
Scallions
Strawberries
Tomatoes
Yellow squash
Zucchini

ALL HERBS & SPICES

FOODS I AVOID:

MEATS TO SKIP

Meat substitutes such as tofu and seitan	Sausages and hot dogs with fillers	Tofu

DAIRY TO SKIP

Milk and any other low-fat dairy products
(unlike heavy cream, these products are high in the milk sugar known as lactose; all milk is naturally high in sugar and so best to avoid with this plan)
Sweetened alternative milks

NUTS & SEEDS TO SKIP

Cashews	Chestnuts	Pistachios

FRUITS & VEGETABLES TO SKIP

Apples	Eggplant	Plantains
Apricots	Grapes	Plums
Artichokes	Honeydew	Potatoes
Bananas	Kiwi	Prunes
Butternut squash	Leeks	Raisins
Cantaloupe	Mangoes	Sweet potatoes
Cherries	Oranges	Turnips
Chickpeas	Parsnips	Water chestnuts
Corn	Peaches	Yams
Dates	Peas	
Edamame	Pineapples	

BEANS & GRAINS

Skip 'em all: No beans, no grains. You won't miss 'em after I'm through with you.

Pantry essentials to have on hand

It's good to have a well-stocked pantry when you are running a Keto kitchen. Buy the best quality of these products that you can, because eating a diet high in fat means you'll want to get the very best forms of these items:

MYRON'S BASIC BBQ KETO SHOPPING LIST

Almonds

Avocados

Bacon
(uncured, which means no added sugar)

Blackberries
(or another low sugar fruit, as you need to have healthy snacks on hand)

Butter
(buy the grass-fed variety if you can)

Cream cheese
(full fat)

Eggs
(pasture-raised, if you can)

Garlic

Greens
(spinach, kale, arugula, etc.)

Heavy cream
or coconut milk

Meats
(grass-fed, if you can)

Olive oil

Sour cream
(full fat)

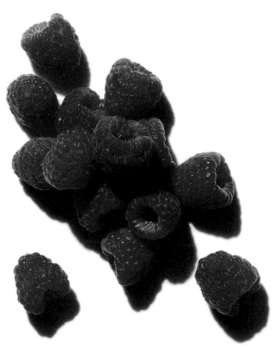

Myron's BBQ Keto Cooking Rules

1. **BUY THE BEST INGREDIENTS YOU CAN AFFORD TO BUY:** I always say this about meats, and it's true. You should cook with the best products you can afford. For Keto barbecuing, you also need to keep in mind that low-quality products might also have more questionable ingredients in them.

2. **CLEAN OUT YOUR PANTRY:** Give away your carb-heavy treats and snacks. Get them out of your house.

3. **KEEP YOUR COOKING SIMPLE:** Stick to recipes like mine that use real food and not a ton of other ingredients. Remember: One of the reasons to choose Keto is that it's supposed to be simple to follow, so keep it easy.

4. **TRACK YOUR FOOD.** No, you don't have to use some fancy kind of macronutrient calculator, but use an app or a notebook. If your memory is good, you can rely on it to keep track of what you put in your mouth. It'll keep you accountable.

5. **PLAN YOUR MEALS.** Prep ingredients ahead of time, know what you're going to eat in advance, and make sure your fridge and pantry are stocked with staples—when your carb cravings hit, you gotta be prepared with other delicious options.

6. **MAKE EXTRA SMOKED MEATS SO YOU CAN PREP AND STORE THEM FOR FUTURE MEALS.** The better you plan ahead, the easier this diet will be. That means cooking in bulk, which is what smoking and barbecuing are all about.

7. **COMMIT.** It takes about a month to fully adapt to a new routine. Keto is meant to be a long-term way of eating, so give yourself time to settle in, adjust, and keep going if you fall off the wagon. Whatever you do, don't give up on yourself. This plan works.

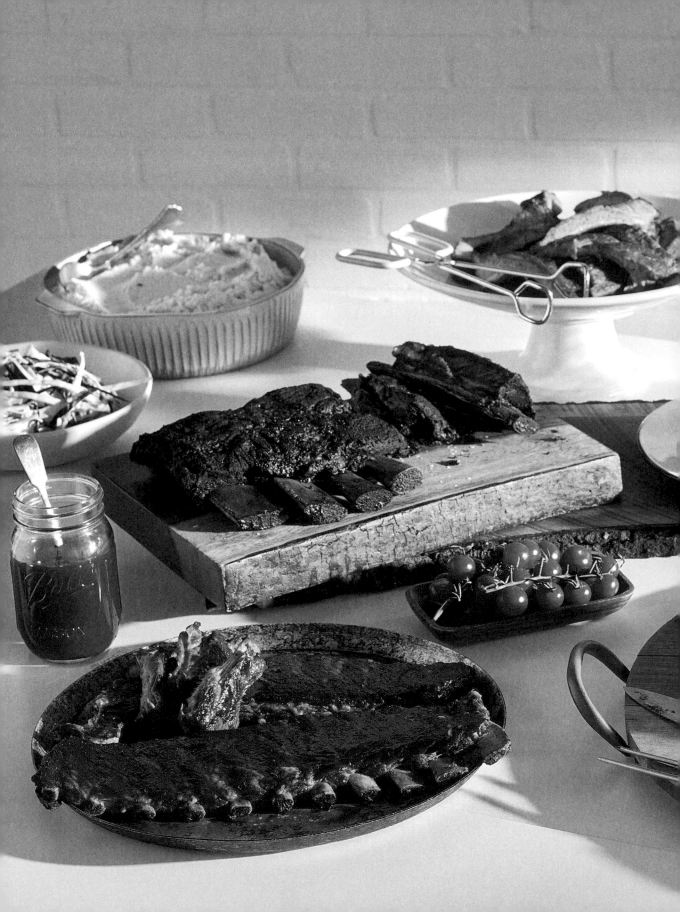

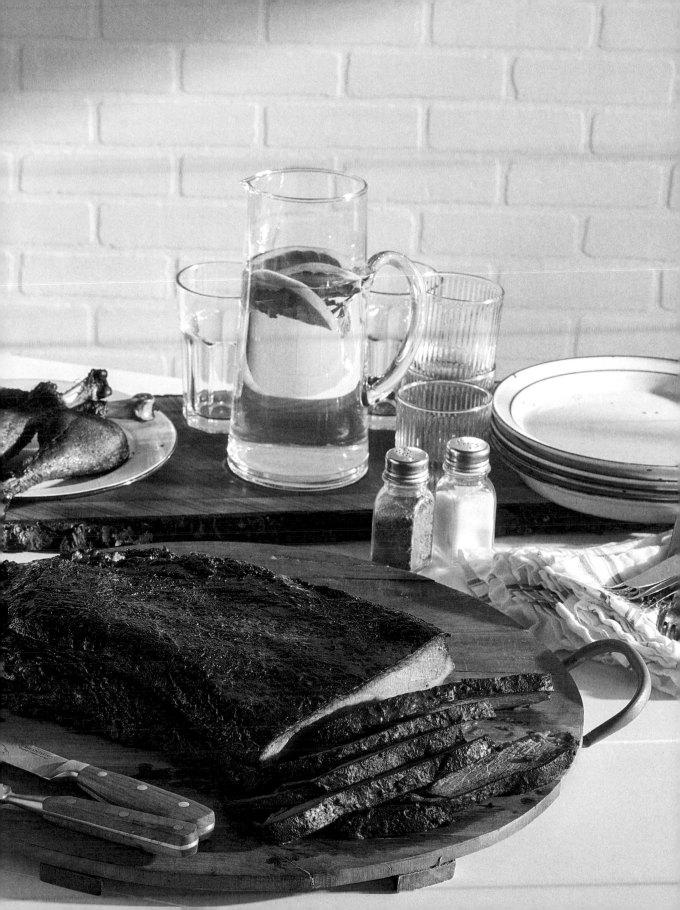

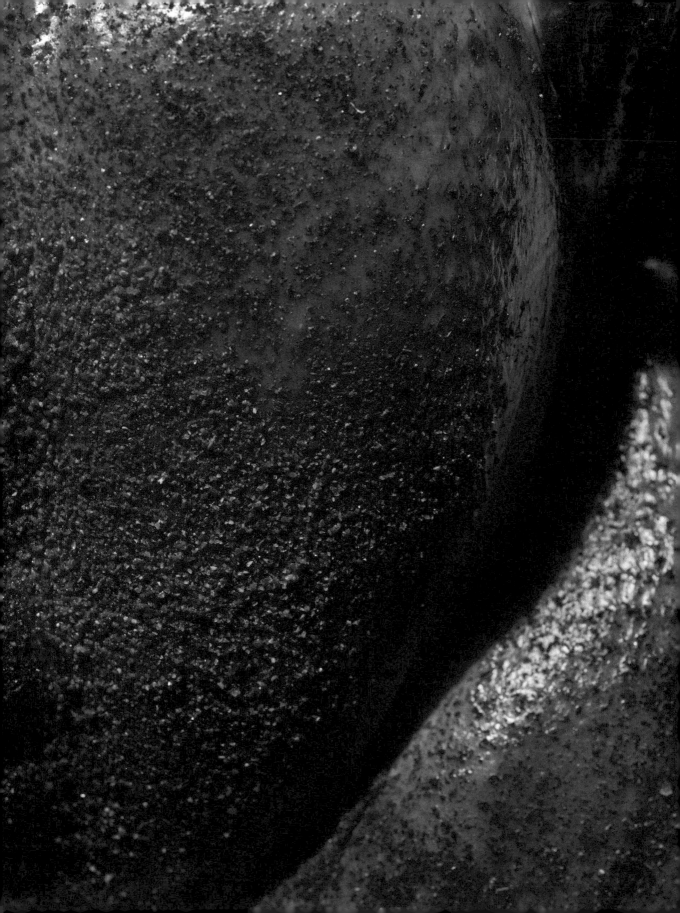

CHAPTER 2

Chicken
and Other Birds

FOR THOSE OF YOU OUT THERE WHO KNOW ME, AND, HELL, LOVE ME—you already know I'm the winningest man in barbecue and I don't need to remind you about it. If you've been following me even for a short amount of time, though, you probably know that chicken used to be what I loved to eat but hated to cook. That was true especially in my early days of cooking in barbecue contests. In those days, I considered chicken the toughest category in competitive barbecue. Why? Because compared to cooking hogs, it involves a lot of tedious prep time to get it organized. The reason it took so long to prepare chicken is because of how barbecue judging works: The pieces had to be absolutely uniform in shape and color, and that's just tough to pull off for a cook—it doesn't matter if all the chicken thighs you cook are not the same exact size when you're eating them in backyard, but in a barbecue competition it'll cost you big points.

I mastered cooking chicken in competitions with "cupcake chicken." Those of you who follow me know this story all too well by now, but if you don't, here's the short version: I created a way to make my chicken thighs uniform, tender and moist by cooking them in a silicon cupcake pan with holes in the bottom, which I've had made custom for me and are sold on my website. That won me a lot of competitions. But my next challenge with chicken was just as hard to figure out how to master: enjoy chicken on my new Keto diet.

Now, chicken is fine according to the Keto diet, but there are some caveats. Number one, there's nothing more boring in the world than a plain old grilled boneless skinless chicken breast. I knew I could not resort to what I've seen lots of dieters—not nearly all of them Keto, mind you—do, which is eat so much plain dry grilled boneless skinless chicken that they eventually go running back to eating unhealthy food. I knew I needed a healthier approach to cooking chicken and other birds like a real pitmaster does, but Keto style. No boring chicken recipes allowed here! What follows are my favorites, my tried-and-true chicken and turkey dishes that keep my body in ketosis, my belly full, and my palate satisfied with tasty flavors.

RECESIPES

BBQ Chicken Rub

MAKES ABOUT 1¾ CUPS

I've had students in my barbecue cooking schools and demos ask me why I make different rubs for different meats. The reason is because the meats themselves have different flavors, so there should not be a one-size-fits-all rub. Chicken is mild and a little sweet, and you can bring out its gentle flavor with a rub that has only a little sweetener (as you know, I like monk fruit sweetener; see page 19 for my notes on why), a little hint of heat (from the cayenne), and the savory hit from the combination of garlic and onion powders. Even if you just sprinkle this rub on your boring boneless skinless chicken breast before you grill it, you're upping your game.

INGREDIENTS

⅔ cup chili powder

2 tablespoons monk fruit sweetener

4 tablespoons kosher salt

¼ cup onion powder

¼ cup garlic powder

1 teaspoon cayenne pepper

1. Combine all the ingredients in a medium bowl or jar. If using a bowl, stir thoroughly to combine, use how much you need, and save the rest for another use. If using a jar, twist the lid on airtight, shake it to mix. You can store this rub in an airtight container, away from heat and light, for up to 6 months.

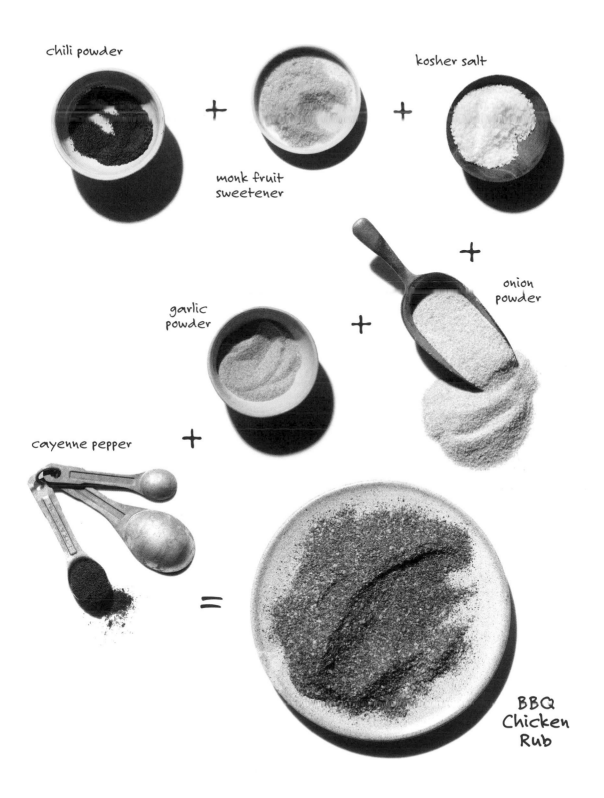

chili powder

+

monk fruit
sweetener

+

kosher salt

+

garlic
powder

+

onion
powder

+

cayenne pepper

=

BBQ
Chicken
Rub

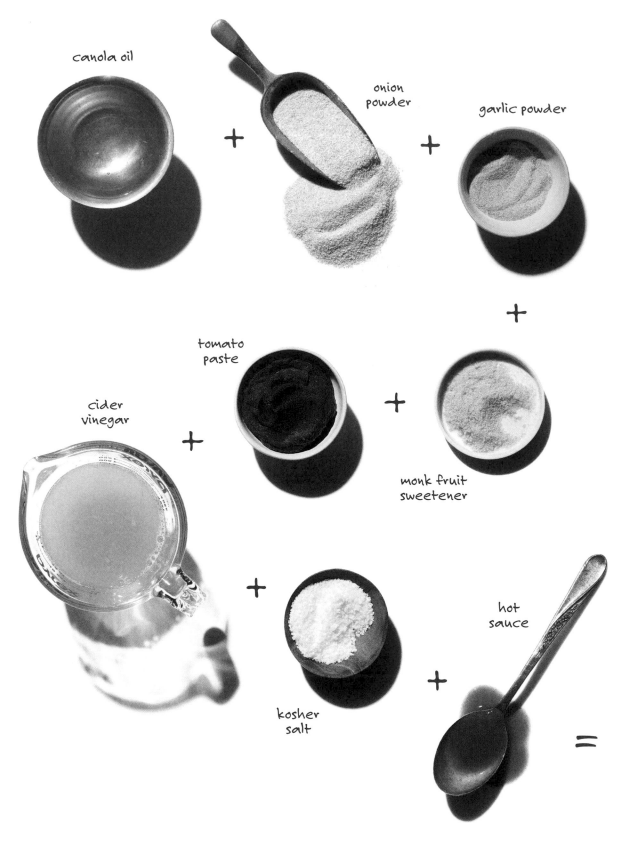

canola oil

+

onion powder

+

garlic powder

+

cider vinegar

+

tomato paste

+

monk fruit sweetener

+

kosher salt

+

hot sauce

=

Tangy Sweet BBQ Sauce

MAKES ABOUT 2 CUPS

I've said it before and I'll say it again: No matter what, good barbecue should let the essential flavor of the meat come through. And just like with rubs and seasonings, sauces come in many varieties and they're not all the same. For my chicken, I like a sauce that has a little more body and a little less bite than the sauce I prefer for hogs. For chicken, whether the meat is light or dark, you need a balanced sauce that helps lock in some flavor and some moisture. That's how to get your chicken to sing!

INGREDIENTS

2 tablespoons canola
or other neutral oil

1 tablespoon onion powder

1 tablespoon garlic powder

2 teaspoons monk fruit sweetener
(*see page 19*)

One 6-ounce can tomato paste

¾ cup cider vinegar

1 teaspoon kosher salt

1 teaspoon hot sauce

1. In a medium saucepan over medium-high heat, warm the oil. Once it's warm, add the other ingredients and stir to combine thoroughly. Cook over medium-low heat, stirring occasionally, until the sauce has slightly thickened, about 15 minutes. Use sauce to baste chicken or top pulled chicken. Leftover sauce may be stored in an airtight jar or other container, refrigerated, for up to 2 months. Always reheat this sauce before using.

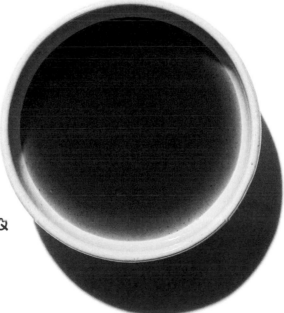

Tangy
Sweet BBQ
Sauce

Smoked Whole Chicken

SERVES 4 TO 6

Even before I was on Keto, I never liked my barbecue chicken to be too saucy or too sweet—a problem I've run into in many barbecue restaurants in my life. I like traditional old-school barbecue chicken, by which I mean a bird that's dry-rubbed, without sauce. This is my personal favorite way to smoke a chicken, and it happens to be the simplest. I sometimes serve chickens this way at my cook schools to introduce my students to the pleasures of plain simple barbecue, of meat that's gently spiced and kissed with smoke. If you're new to smoking, this is probably the single best recipe to get yourself started cooking. I like to cut the back out of the chicken as it cooks quicker and better, but you can skip that step if you want.

INGREDIENTS

**1 whole chicken
(about 3-4 pounds)**

1 recipe BBQ Chicken Rub
(page 30)

OPTIONAL: Tangy Sweet BBQ Sauce
(page 32)

1. Heat a smoker to 250°F.

2. Place whole chicken breast side down on a clean work surface. Using kitchen shears and starting at the thigh end, cut along one side of backbone all the way up past the neck bottom. From the other side of the backbone, cut all the way up again and remove the backbone. Discard or save to make a stock.

3. Use paper towels or a clean kitchen towel to pat the chicken pieces dry thoroughly so that the rub will adhere to the skin. Generously apply the chicken rub all over the exposed areas of the chicken, rubbing it in gently. Place the seasoned chicken in a deep aluminum baking pan. Place the plan in the smoker and cook for 1½ hours.

4. After 3 hours, start checking the internal temperature by inserting the thermometer into the thickest part of the breast without touching bone. When the breast reaches 165°F, remove the pan from the smoker. Allow the chicken to rest, uncovered, for 15 minutes. Serve immediately, with the wings and some warm Tangy Sweet BBQ Sauce on the side, if you like.

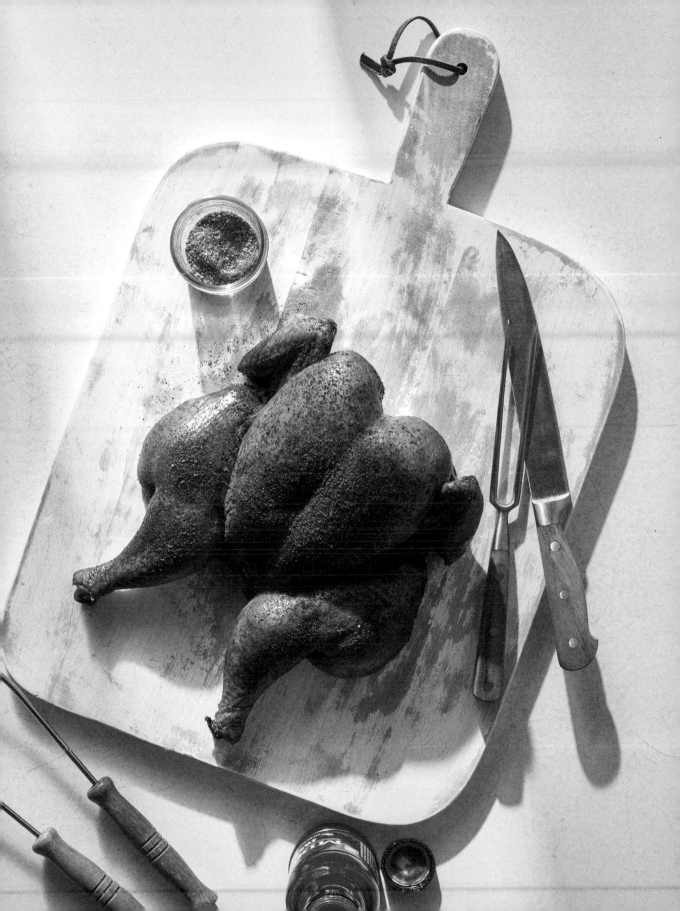

Extra-Crispy Grilled Chicken Thighs

I cannot tell you how often folks ask me about the skin on their chicken thighs—why does it always come out rubbery? they ask. Well, let me tell you: Brushing them with butter, which is a distinctly Keto cooking method, is going to be your best friend here. Try that, then say hello to your new crispy chicken thighs.

INGREDIENTS

10 to 12 bone-in chicken thighs

½ cup butter, melted

1 tablespoon salt

2 teaspoons black pepper

¼ cup BBQ Chicken Rub (*page 30*)

1. Light the grill. Brush the thighs all over with half of the melted butter, reserving ¼ cup. Generously season the thighs with the salt, pepper, and rub. Grill over moderately high heat, basting with the remaining butter, until just done, about 12 minutes per side.

BBQ Bacon-Wrapped Chicken Breasts

I know the stereotype about the Keto diet, the one that says that people go on it just for the excuse of eating pounds and pounds of bacon. Well, I do not eat pounds and pounds of bacon. In fact, you'd be surprised to learn that once you can have all the bacon you want, you find that you don't need to indulge in it all the time. That said, wrapping a chicken breast in bacon gives it some delicious extra smoky flavor (remember that the extra fat is absolutely permitted on Keto—you need it to keep your body in ketosis). So, you know, here's where to put some extra bacon if you want it.

INGREDIENTS

4 large boneless skinless chicken breasts

1 cup Tangy Sweet BBQ Sauce (*page 32*)

1 medium white onion, diced

3 cloves garlic, crushed

1 cup BBQ Chicken Rub (*page 30*)

8 thin slices bacon

1. Place the chicken breasts in a shallow dish or large plastic bag, and add the barbecue sauce, onion, and garlic. Mix to coat. Cover or seal and refrigerate overnight.

2. When ready to cook, preheat the smoker to 325°F.

3. Remove the chicken from the marinade, shaking off the excess sauce, and apply the rub liberally to each breast. Wrap each breast in two slices of the bacon, securing the slices with toothpicks. Place the breasts in a large aluminum baking pan. Place the pan in the smoker and cook the breasts for 1 hour, or until their internal temperature reaches 165°F.

4. Remove the pan from the smoker and let the breasts rest, uncovered, in the pan for 15 minutes. Then slice the breasts and serve with extra Tangy Sweet BBQ Sauce on the side for dipping, if you like.

WINGS TWO WAYS
Smoked Wings

MAKES 24 PIECES

I announce to all my cooking classes that I am a wing man. Chicken wings are my favorite appetizer, and that's a fact. I love everything about 'em, particularly that it's considered perfectly acceptable in any public place to pick them up and eat them with your hands. I like my wings all ways, with just about any kind of sauce or flavoring you can think of cooking them with. That said, when I started Keto I had to figure out how to make them without coating them in flour and frying them. Guess what? It wasn't that hard. Here are my favorite preparations. God bless wings.

INGREDIENTS

12 whole chicken wings, or 24 drumettes and flats

1 cup BBQ Chicken Rub (*page 30*)

2 cups Tangy Sweet BBQ Sauce (*page 32*)

1. Heat a smoker to 250°F.

2. If using whole wings: Use a sharp knife to cut each wing in half to separate the flats from the drumettes.

3. Apply the rub liberally to each wing. Place the wings in an aluminum baking pan in a single layer. Place the pan in the smoker and cook, uncovered, for 2 hours.

4. Remove the pan from the smoker, brush the Tangy Sweet BBQ Sauce all over the wings, and return the pan to the smoker. Cook uncovered for an additional 15 minutes. Remove the pan from the smoker and eat immediately, with extra sauce on the side for dipping if you like.

How to Separate a Chicken Wing

You can buy chicken wings already separated into pieces, but it's also easy to do it yourself. Chicken wings have two joints: One connects the wing tip to the forearm (or "flat" as wings fans know it) and the other connects the foreman or flat to the upper arm (or "drumette"). First: find both joints. Second: use a sharp knife to cut right through the hinge of each joint. I put my hand on the flat part of my knife to bear straight down and push hard rather than sawing the blade back and forth across the joint.

WINGS TWO WAYS
Buffalo Keto Wings

INGREDIENTS

¼ cup Tangy Sweet BBQ Sauce
(*page 32*)

¼ cup hot sauce

1 tablespoon plus 2 teaspoons
unsalted butter, melted

12 whole chicken wings,
or 24 drumettes and flats

*OPTIONAL: Blue Cheese Dressing
(page 164), Pitmaster's Buttermilk
Ranch Dressing (page 163)*

1. In a large bowl, combine the barbecue sauce, hot sauce, and melted butter. Set aside.

2. If using whole wings: Use a sharp knife to cut each wing in half to separate the flats from the drumettes.

3. Place the wings in a large plastic bag or bowl, cover with ½ the sauce, and toss to coat. Reserve the remaining sauce. Seal or cover and let the wings marinate for 20 to 30 minutes. (This can also be done overnight; the butter sauce will congeal a bit, but that's fine.)

4. When you are ready to cook the wings, heat the broiler. Shake excess marinade from the wings and then transfer them to either a rimmed baking sheet lined with aluminum foil or an aluminum baking pan, taking care to arrange them in a single layer spaced a little apart. Discard the marinade.

5. Broil the wings for 10 to 12 minutes. Flip the wings over and broil until the skin is crispy and the meat pulls easily from the bones, about 10 minutes more.

6. Toss wings with the reserved sauce mixture, coating each one thoroughly. Serve wings piping hot with Blue Cheese Dressing or Pitmaster's Buttermilk Ranch Dressing on the side, if you like.

Pulled Smoked Chicken Two Ways

MAKES 5 TO 7 CUPS COOKED CHICKEN

The first thing you've got to do here is smoke a chicken. Here's my suggestion: Smoke two of 'em at the same time. Eat the first one for your dinner. Let the second one cool completely, pull all the meat off it, and use it another day in other meals. You can get about 6 cups of chicken off a 4 pound roasted chicken, and the ratio of white to dark meat with that will be 2:1. For my smoked pulled chicken, I like to mix the light and dark meat together, but you should do as you please. Here are two ways you can use that great smoked chicken meat.

INGREDIENTS

2 cups chicken broth

⅓ cup monk fruit sweetener (*see page 19*)

1 chicken (about 3½ pounds), cut into 8 pieces

2 cups Tangy Sweet BBQ Sauce (*page 32*)

1½ cups (3 sticks) unsalted butter, at room temperature

1. In a large bowl, combine the broth with the sweetener; stir well to dissolve the sweetener. Place the chicken pieces in the mixture and marinate, covered in the refrigerator, for at least 4 hours and preferably overnight.

2. When you are ready to cook the chicken, heat a smoker to 250°F.

3. Remove the chicken from the marinade and shake off excess. Apply the rub liberally to all the pieces. Place the pieces, skin-side up, in a deep aluminum baking pan. Rub the chicken pieces all over with the butter; if any butter remains, place it in the plan with the chicken. Place the pan in the smoker and cook for 30 minutes.

4. Remove the pan from the smoker, flip the chicken pieces so they are skin-side down, and return the pan to the smoker. Cook for 1 hour or until the internal temperature of the chicken reaches 155°F.

5. Remove the pan from the smoker and sprinkle a little more rub over the chicken. Return it to the smoker and cook for 15 minutes.

6. Remove the pan from the smoker and brush the chicken sauce over the pieces. Return it to the smoker for another 15 minutes to let the sauce soak into the chicken.

7. Remove the pan from the smoker and let the chicken rest, uncovered, to cool to room temperature, for about 20 minutes. Use your fingers or the tines of two forks to gently "pull" the chicken meat from the bones. Then shred the chicken into thin strips, discarding any excess fat, cartilage, and bones as you go. Serve it in one of the following ways:

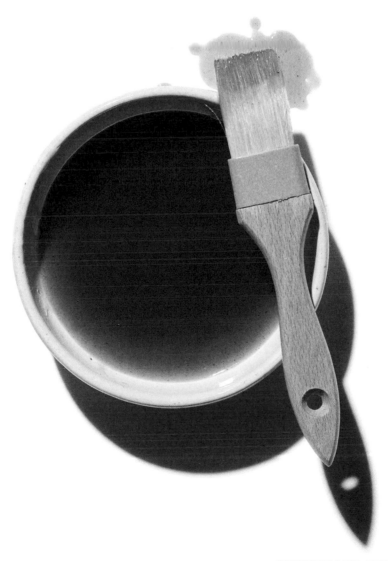

PULLED SMOKED CHICKEN TWO WAYS
Pulled Chicken Keto "Sandwiches"

After you pull your chicken, it'll take you no more than 15 minutes to make these wraps—and that's if you're moving slow. I count on each person eating about ½ cup of pulled chicken, but how much you put on each lettuce wrap depends on you. You can use any kind of Keto bread you like in place of these wraps, but I prefer to enjoy them like this.

INGREDIENTS

2 cups Pulled Smoked Chicken (*page 40*)

⅓ cup Tangy Sweet BBQ Sauce (*page 32*)

½ large head iceberg lettuce, core removed, head quartered

¼ red onion, sliced very thin

1. In a medium bowl toss the chicken in the sauce.

2. Pile pulled chicken on lettuce leaves. Drizzle sauce on top of the chicken and top with red onion slices, wrapping the lettuce around the fillings. You can add any number of toppings to these sandwich wraps, including diced bacon or avocados, sprigs of cilantro, or shredded cheddar cheese.

PULLED SMOKED CHICKEN TWO WAYS
Pulled Chicken "Sandwich Bowls"

MAKES 2 "SANDWICH BOWLS"

A lot of folks like me on the Keto eating plan have come up with clever ways to enjoy sandwiches without carbs. Sandwich bowls are one of my favorites, as you basically take your favorite ingredients for sandwiches, get rid of the bread, and turn them into what seems like an even bigger meal. Smoked pulled chicken works perfectly for a BBQ version of a healthy bowl.

INGREDIENTS

2 cups romaine lettuce hearts, chopped

6 slices provolone cheese, cut into thin slices

3 pickles, cut into thin slices

4 banana peppers, cut into rings

1 bell pepper, cut into strips

6 cherry tomatoes

⅓ cup olive oil

2 tablespoons red wine vinegar

1 teaspoon Italian seasoning

2 cups Pulled Smoked Chicken (*page 40*)

OPTIONAL: salt, pepper, and Tangy Sweet BBQ Sauce (page 32)

1. Combine the lettuce, cheese, pickles, peppers, and tomatoes in a large bowl.

2. In a small bowl whisk together the olive oil, vinegar, and Italian seasoning just to combine. Immediately dress the veggies in the bowl. Let sit for 10 minutes so the veggies can absorb the dressing.

3. Divide the vegetables between two large salad bowls or plates. Mound 1 cup of pulled chicken on top of each. If you'd like, season with salt and pepper and Tangy Sweet BBQ Sauce.

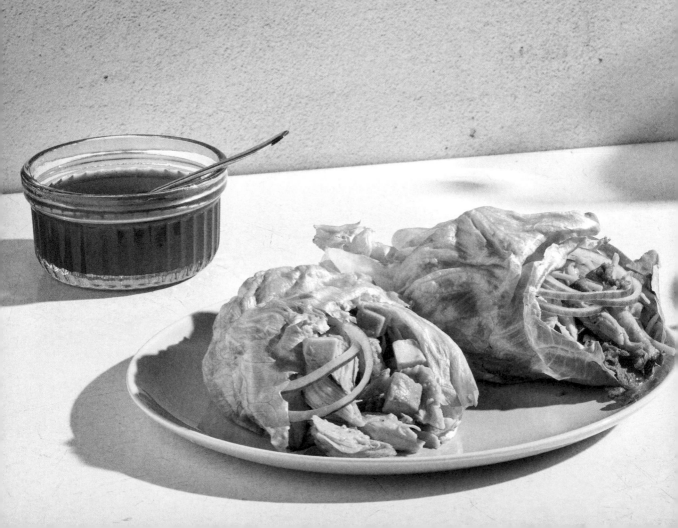

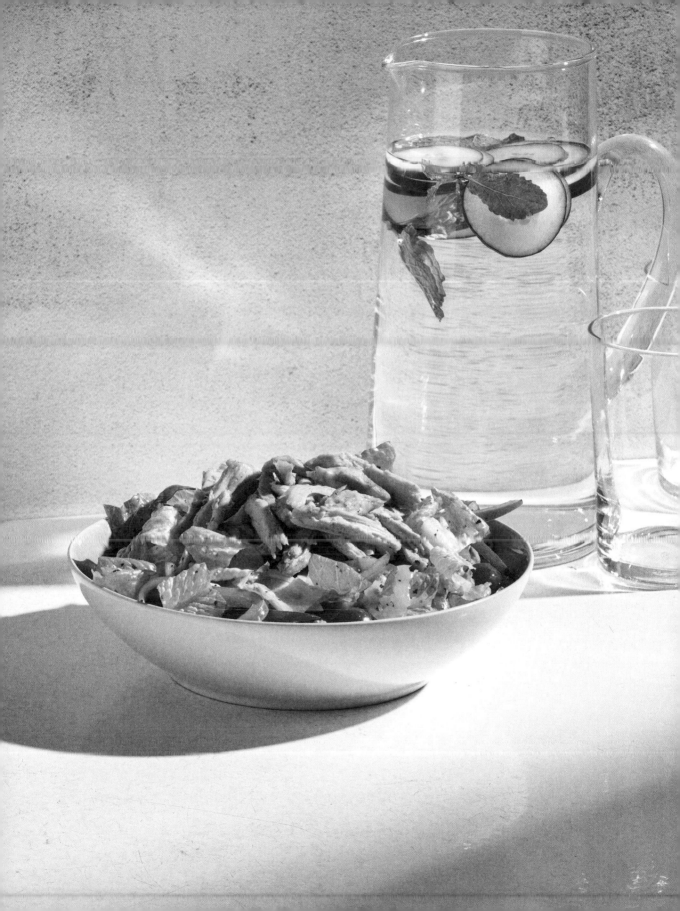

Southern "Fried" Chicken Tenders

SERVES 2 TO 4

All my friends and family know that fried chicken is probably my favorite food of all time. I grew up on it. I love it. When I committed to the Keto diet, I had to figure out how I could still enjoy this Southern classic. Believe what I'm preaching: It's not that challenging to adapt your favorite recipes to fit this eating plan. For example, substituting crushed pork rinds in place of flour creates a flavorful crunchy coating. It's so crunchy, in fact, that I don't even have to bother with the messy fuss (not to mention the unhealthiness) of deep-frying these bad boys.

INGREDIENTS

½ cup buttermilk

Hot sauce (I prefer Louisiana style)

2 large whole boneless skinless chicken breasts, cut into strips

6 ounces of pork rinds

2 teaspoons kosher salt

1 teaspoon black pepper

½ teaspoon garlic powder

½ teaspoon smoked paprika

1 egg

¼ cup mayonnaise

¼ cup Dijon mustard

OPTIONAL: ½ cup Tangy Sweet BBQ Sauce (page 32)

1. Pour the buttermilk into a large plastic bag, add a few dashes of hot sauce, add the chicken strips, seal the bag airtight, and massage it around a few minutes to coat all the chicken, then let it marinate in the refrigerator for at least 20 minutes. You can leave them in the fridge like this overnight if you want to, but not much longer than that.

2. When you're ready to cook the chicken, preheat your oven to 400°F.

3. Line a large baking sheet with parchment paper or coat it with cooking spray, and then set it aside.

4. Put the pork rinds in a small plastic bag. Use a rolling pin or a measuring cup or your own fist to crush them until they become crumbs. Pour the crumbs into a bowl and stir in the salt, pepper, garlic powder, and paprika.

5. In a separate bowl, beat together the egg with the mayonnaise and mustard.

recipe continues

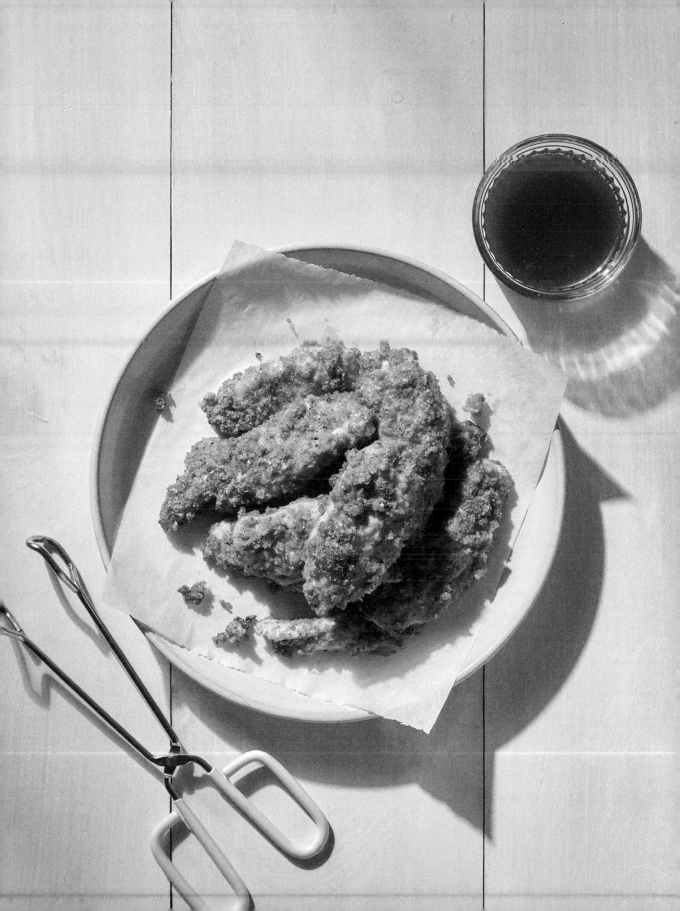

6. Remove all the chicken strips from the bag and discard the marinade. Pat the chicken strips dry with paper towels. To bread each chicken strip: First lay it in the pork rind crumbs, turn it to coat, then use tongs or a fork to dunk it into the egg batter, swirling to coat. Finally, dredge the chicken back through the pork rinds, pressing it down gently but firmly to make sure the crumbs stick. Transfer the chicken tender to the baking pan. Repeat the process until all the chicken tenders are coated.

7. Spray the tenders with cooking spray, then bake for about 20 minutes or until the tenders are golden brown.

8. If you'd like, serve with Tangy Sweet BBQ Sauce for dipping.

Grilled Bacon-Wrapped Chicken Livers

This is a great example of an answer to the question my fans ask me when they want to know what I like to eat at home. I love these suckers and think they're just about the perfect appetizer to go with my cocktail. I've talked about these so much that one time, a guy at a competition I was cooking in came up and told me that I got him hooked on them. He had fired up his smoker just to make some chicken livers. That's how much he loves them. That might be too much. I make these when I'm already smoking something else, so you get the most use from your smoker and from your time cooking on it as possible. In other words, this is a great add-on when you're already smoking a piece of meat.

INGREDIENTS

8 ounces bacon

1 pound chicken livers

1 cup BBQ Chicken Rub (*page 30*)

1 cup Tangy Sweet BBQ Sauce (*page 32*)

1. Heat a smoker to 325°F.

2. Cut the bacon slices in half crosswise. Set them aside.

3. Rinse the chicken livers thoroughly in fresh cold water, and then use paper towels or a clean kitchen towel to pat them dry. Lightly prick each one with a fork to prevent it from popping open. Sprinkle the livers all over with the rub. Wrap each liver in a bacon strip, securing it with a toothpick. Transfer the wrapped chicken liver to a medium-size aluminum pan. Repeat the process with the rest of the livers and bacon.

4. Place the pan in the smoker and cook for approximately 10 minutes, or until the bacon is thoroughly cooked. Remove the pan from the smoker and use a brush to glaze the livers with the sauce. Serve and enjoy while hot.

White Chili with Smoked Chicken

SERVES 4 TO 6

Let me be honest with you: Not every single recipe translates to Keto. My beloved Brunswick stew, which is a native of Georgia just like I am, contains corn, and you have to make a roux with flour to make a good version. Instead of trying to adapt that to Keto, I decided to work on a hearty chili recipe that would be rich and filling but allow me to stay on my plan. If you think you've had white chili with chicken before, I can promise you that it's much, much more delicious when you make it with smoked chicken. I still love Brunswick stew and I allow myself to have it as an occasional treat, but this chili is a staple.

INGREDIENTS

2 tablespoons butter

1 teaspoon olive oil

1 large onion, diced

1 bell pepper, seeded and chopped

1 jalapeño pepper, seeded and chopped

4 gloves garlic, minced

2 cups Pulled Smoked Chicken (*page 40*)

1 tablespoon salt

1 tablespoon ground cumin

1 teaspoon coriander

4 cups chicken broth

14 ounces chopped green chiles

¼ cup heavy cream

¼ cup cream cheese

OPTIONAL: chopped scallions, grated cheddar cheese, chopped crisp bacon, BBQ Chicken Rub (page 30)

1. In a large pot over medium-high heat, heat the butter and let it melt but not foam or smoke. Add the olive oil, onion, peppers, jalapeños, and garlic. Sauté to soften, about 3 minutes, but do not let the vegetables brown. Turn down the heat to medium. Add the chicken, salt, and spices. Toss with the veggies to coat. Slowly pour in the broth, green chiles, cream, and cream cheese. Stir to incorporate the cream cheese fully. Lower the heat to medium-low and let simmer, covered for 30 minutes.

2. Serve warm, and if you'd like, garnished with scallions, cheddar cheese, bacon, and/or BBQ Chicken Rub.

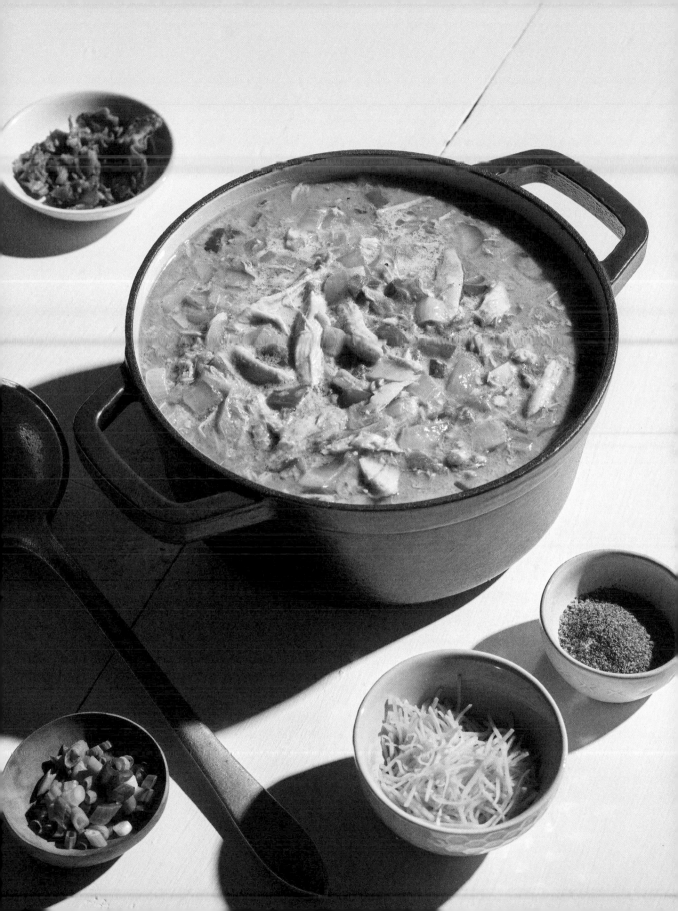

Whole Smoked Turkey

This recipe pretty much answers the question I get about what I eat on Keto at Thanksgiving. Answer: I smoke a turkey like I always do. Following the BBQ Keto lifestyle, I just cut out the side dishes with tons of carbs and sugar.

INGREDIENTS

8 cups chicken broth

3 medium white onions, diced

4 garlic cloves, crushed

⅓ cup monk fruit sweetener (*see page 19*)

1 12- to 15-pound turkey, neck and giblets removed

2 cups BBQ Chicken Rub (*page 30*)

1. In a very large mixing bowl, combine the chicken broth, onions, garlic, and monk fruit sweetener.

2. Place the turkey in a large plastic brining/marinating bag or clean and sanitized cooler, and poor the broth mixture over it. Tie the bag to seal it well, place in refrigerator (or a cooler with enough ice to keep cool overnight), and allow the turkey to marinate overnight.

3. When you are ready to cook the turkey, heat a smoker to 250°F.

4. Remove the turkey from the marinade and discard the marinade. Using paper towels or a clean kitchen towel, pat the turkey dry all over. Apply the rub all over the bird, inside and out, hitting every available surface. Transfer the turkey into a large, deep aluminum pan that will hold it snugly, then place the pan in the smoker. Cook the turkey for about 5 hours, or until the breast meat reaches an internal temperature of 165°F.

5. Remove the turkey from the smoker. Allow the turkey to rest, loosely covered with foil, for 30 minutes. Then carve the turkey and serve immediately.

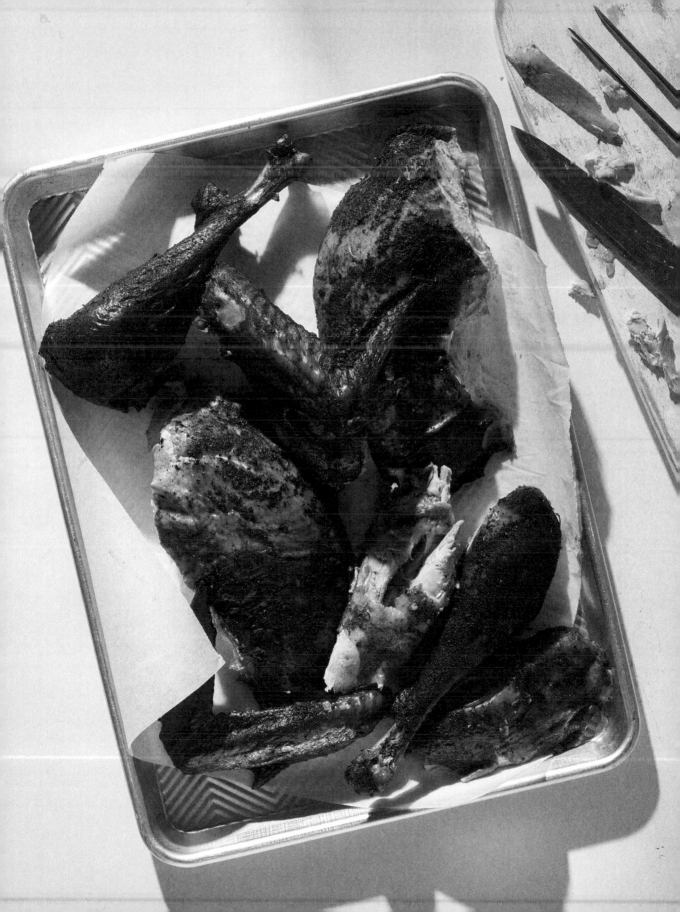

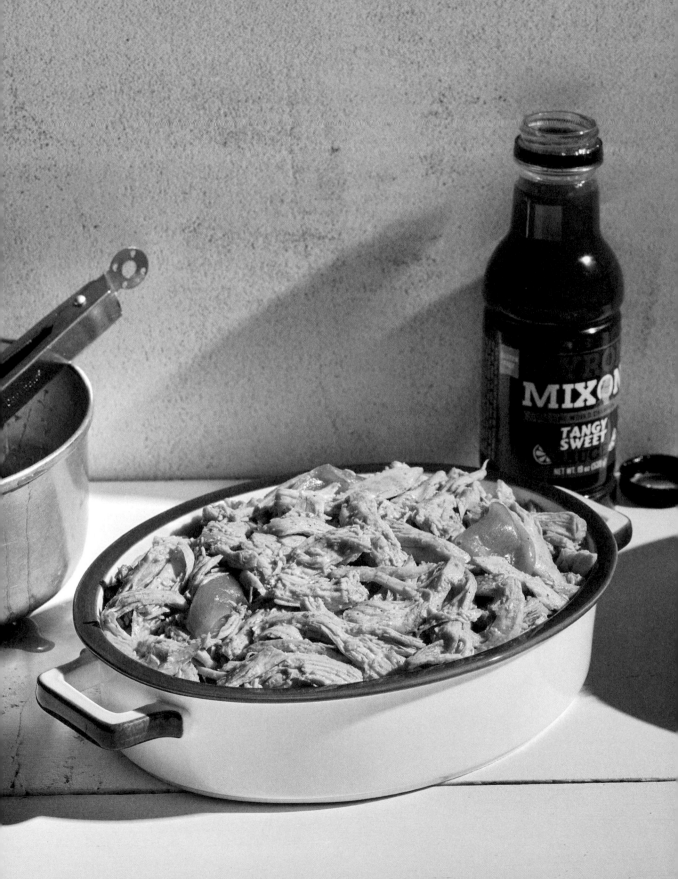

Slow Cooker Pulled Turkey

SERVES 6

This is one sure-fire way to get a tender, juicy turkey breast infused with barbecue flavors. In addition to eating the pulled turkey as a main course, you can use it to fill bowls, build lettuce wraps, or to top a salad. It's just good stuff to have around when those of us on the Keto plan get hungry. All you need to make it is a 6-quart slow cooker and a good appetite.

INGREDIENTS

1 bone-in skin-on whole turkey breast (5 to 6 pounds)

½ cup (1 stick) butter, at room temperature

½ cup BBQ Chicken Rub (*page 30*)

3 medium white onions, quartered

12 garlic cloves, peeled

½ cup Tangy Sweet BBQ Sauce (*page 32*)

1. Using a clean kitchen towel or paper towels, pat the breast dry. Slowly work your fingers under the skin of the breast to separate it from the meat. Take care not to tear the skin. Gently push the butter under the skin, rubbing it over the meat so that it's covered completely and evenly coats the meat. Put rub on the outside skin and pat (don't rub) it in.

2. Arrange the onions and garlic cloves in the bottom of a 6-quart slow cooker. Place the turkey breast on top of the onions and garlic and set the slow cooker to low. Cook until the breast is moist, tender, and falls apart when prodded with a fork; 6 to 8 hours depending on the size of the breast.

3. Remove the breast from the slow cooker and separate the breast meat from the bone. Place the turkey back in the slow cooker with any accumulated juices, onions, and garlic. Use two forks to shred the turkey breast in the juices. Transfer the pulled turkey to a bowl. Toss with Tangy Sweet BBQ Sauce. Serve however you'd like.

Smoked Sausage-Stuffed Turkey Breast

SERVES 10 TO 12

One thing people don't know about me is that even though I'm known for being the world's best pitmaster, I also know some sophisticated cooking techniques. I'm a well-rounded chef—just not as round as I used to be! I like stuffing meats for variety and flavor, and a turkey breast, which is lean and subtly flavored, is just about the perfect thing to stuff with some rich, flavorful, herby, salty pork sausage. I add some Georgia pecans in there for crunch. Once you taste this, you'll thank me for that addition, too.

INGREDIENTS

½ cup (1 stick) butter

1 small yellow onion, diced

2 stalks celery, diced

8 ounces sweet pork sausage, removed from casing

12 (or so) whole pecans, chopped

Salt and pepper

1 boneless skin-on whole turkey breast, approximately 5 pounds

2 cups Tangy Sweet BBQ Sauce (*page 32*)

1. First make the sausage stuffing: In a large pan over medium heat, melt the butter until hot but not foaming or smoking. Add the onions and celery and sauté gently until the vegetables become translucent; do not brown. Add the sausage to the pan. Use a spatula to break it up into crumbles. Cook until the sausage is golden brown. Transfer the sausage to a bowl and stir in the pecans. They will absorb the butter and fat rendered from the sausage. Allow the mixture to cool to room temperature. Season the mixture to your liking with salt and pepper.

2. Meanwhile, butterfly and flatten the turkey breast. Turn the breast over (so the side that had skin is facing down) and lay it flat on a cutting board. Using a sharp chef's knife, slice into the thickest portion of the breast. Cut along the length of the breast, but not all the way through. Unfold so the breast opens like a book. Cover the entire area with a piece of plastic wrap and pound with a meat mallet until the turkey is of uniform thickness (about ½ inch). Season both sides all over with salt and pepper. Spread the sausage mixture in an even layer all over the surface

of the butterflied breast, leaving about a 1-inch-thick border around all the edges. Starting with one short end, roll into a log, completely enclosing the stuffing. Use kitchen twine to tie the roll; you'll need about 4 or 5 evenly spaced ties to hold it together securely. Transfer the roll to an aluminum pan. You can prep the turkey breast to this stage up to 24 hours before you are ready to cook it, just keep it in the refrigerator until you're ready to cook.

3. Heat a smoker to 375°F.

4. Transfer the pan to the smoker. Cook the turkey breast for about 40 minutes, or until the internal temperature of the thickest part of the breast reaches 160°F. Remove the pan from the smoker. Glaze the turkey breast all over on all sides with the sauce. Put the pan back in the smoker and cook for 10 additional minutes to set the glaze. Remove the pan from the smoker, let the turkey breast rest for 10 minutes, and then slice and serve.

State Fair-Style Smoked Turkey Legs

Welcome to Six Flags Over Georgia, Disneyland, and the Iowa State Fair. These giant smoked drumsticks bring everybody's favorite amusement park treat to your backyard. And the best part is, they're Keto-friendly!

INGREDIENTS

1 gallon water

1 cup kosher salt

2 tablespoons monk fruit sweetener (*see page 19*)

3 tablespoons garlic powder

3 tablespoons onion powder

3 tablespoons dried sage

1 tablespoon smoked paprika

1 tablespoon black pepper

1 teaspoon ground cinnamon

1 teaspoon ground allspice

8 turkey legs

1. In a large stock pot, combine all the ingredients except the turkey legs. Bring to a boil over medium-high heat. Let boil for 2 minutes. Remove the pot from the heat and let the brine cool completely.

2. When the brine has cooled, arrange the turkey legs in a cooler or in several large plastic bags. Pour the brine over the turkey legs, making sure they're completely submerged. Refrigerate the legs in the brine overnight.

3. When you're ready to cook the legs, heat your smoker to 300°F.

4. Transfer the turkey legs to a very large aluminum pan or divide them between 2, making sure they're not right on top of each other. They need a little space between them. Smoke the turkey legs for 3½ to 4 hours or until they are a burnished red-brown and the internal temperature in the thickest part of the leg registers 165°F.

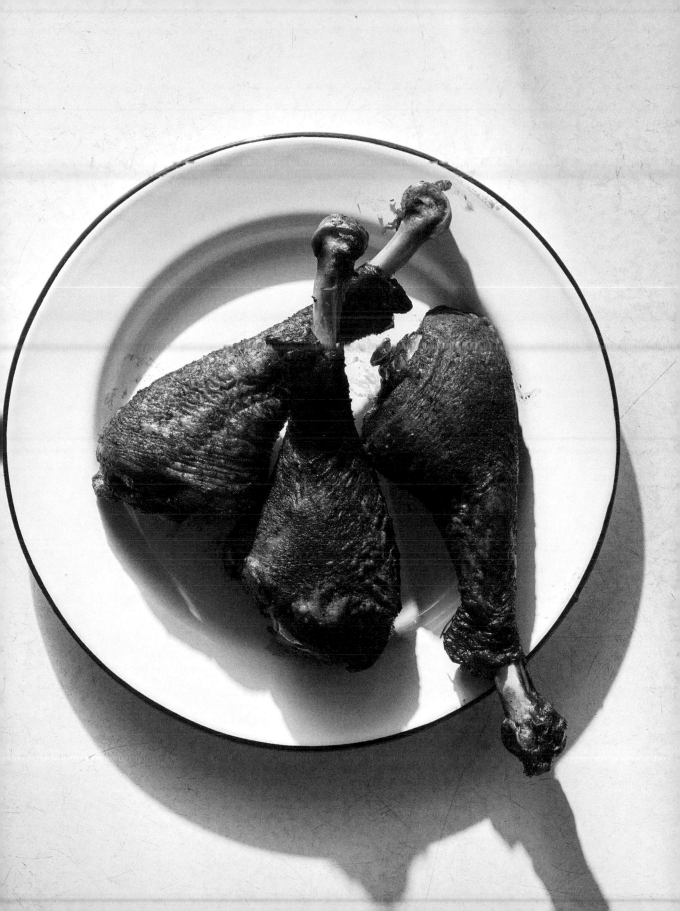

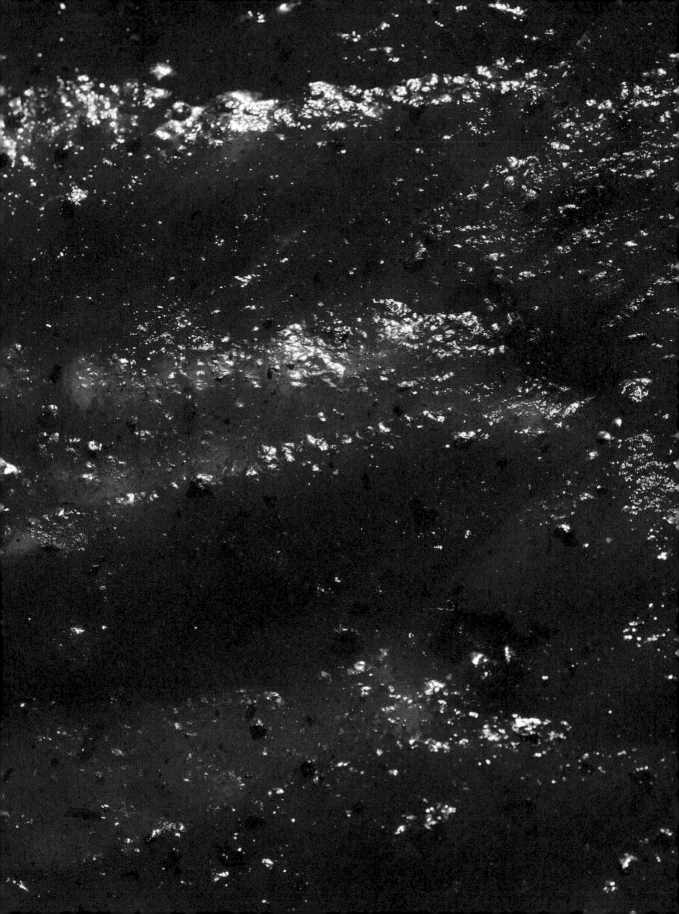

CHAPTER 3

Pork

IT'S ONLY FITTING to begin this chapter of Keto pork recipes by reminding y'all that I'm a four-time competitive barbecue world champion and have been dubbed "The Best Hog Cook in the World."

This is no accident, people. I'm not only a fierce competitor and a perennial winner who stands on podiums and collects trophies (even better: collects checks) at contests. I'm a hog specialist. People like me, which is to say folks who come from one of the ten counties that make up middle Georgia, are familiar with barbecue, and with pork barbecue in particular. Combine where I come from with the fact that my daddy Jack Mixon owned a barbecue take-out business here in Georgia, in our hometown of Vienna (it's pronounced VIE-anna down here).

I spent my childhood shoveling coals into fire barrels to keep my dad's pits going, to keep that hog meat smoking—and that's no exaggeration. My dad was pretty damn tough on us, but it paid off the first time I took first place in a barbecue cooking contest. Yes, in the very first barbecue contest I entered, the Lock & Dam BBQ Contest in Augusta, Georgia, in 1996, I took first place in the whole-hog category; first place in the ribs category; and third place in pork shoulder. And you know what? I'm grateful for my dad's grit and determination to work my butt off shoveling coals, which helped to turn me into a barbecue cook. This is my explanation every time someone asks me how I got to be so good at smoking hogs.

All of this is to say that if I know anything about anything in this life, I know about smoking hogs. Everything about it—the taste of the meat, the tenderness of it, even the appearance of it—is second nature to me. And I'm here to tell you that once you understand a few basic principles, cooking pork can become second nature to you as well. It all boils down to this: Smoked pork should taste full-flavored, tangy, rich, and complex. What does that mean? It means that the best barbecue should taste like meat. Not grape jelly or maple syrup or cherry juice or any other so-called "secret ingredient" that folks say they put in their barbecue sauce. You do not need all that sugary stuff to make your barbecue taste good. What should come through is the deliciously mild flavor of pork kissed with smoke. That's perfection, right there.

In this chapter you'll find a healthful approach to cooking the main event in real Southern BBQ—pork—with an emphasis on techniques that bring out the meat's natural flavor without adding sweeteners, and let you stay on the Keto diet.

RECIPES

THE BASICS:

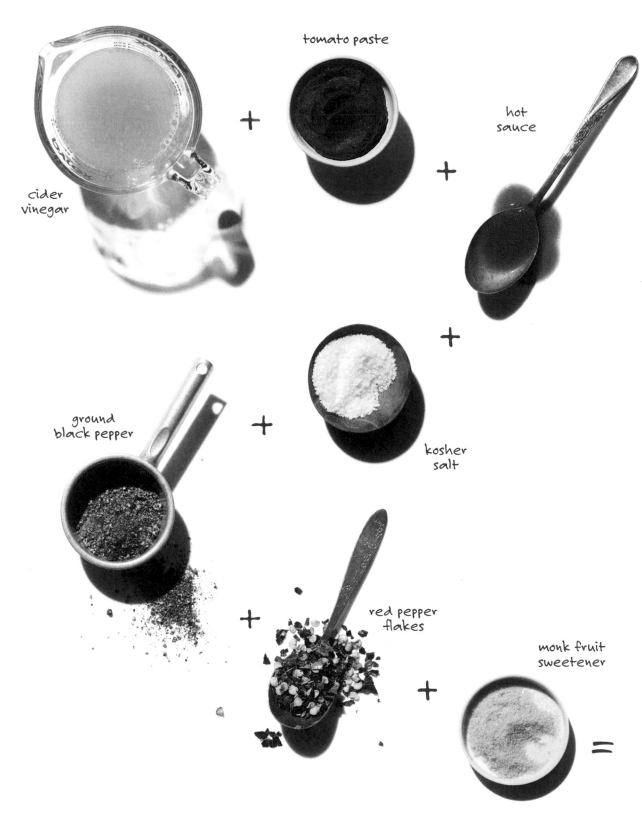

cider
vinegar

tomato paste

hot
sauce

ground
black pepper

kosher
salt

red pepper
flakes

monk fruit
sweetener

=

THE BASICS
Vinegar BBQ Sauce

MAKES ABOUT 3½ CUPS

This is my Keto-friendly version of the classic sauce for pork barbecue that is nearest and dearest to my heart. There's nothing fancy about this sauce. It's designed to allow the essential flavor of the smoked pork to come through with every bite. The flavors cooperate with each other in your mouth and enhance the natural sweetness of the pork without overpowering it.

INGREDIENTS

2 cups cider vinegar

1 cup tomato paste

½ cup hot sauce

2 tablespoons kosher salt

2 tablespoons ground black pepper

1 tablespoon red pepper flakes

1 tablespoon monk fruit sweetener (*see page 19*)

1. In a heavy, medium-sized pot set over medium heat, combine the vinegar, tomato paste, and hot sauce. Stir until well mixed. Add the salt, pepper, and red pepper flakes and stir to dissolve. Stir in the monk fruit sweetener and allow the mixture to come to a simmer but do not let it boil. When the spices are thoroughly dissolved, take the pot off the heat and set aside to cool to room temperature. Funnel the sauce into bottles or containers of your choice. Cover tightly. The sauce will keep, refrigerated, for up to 1 year.

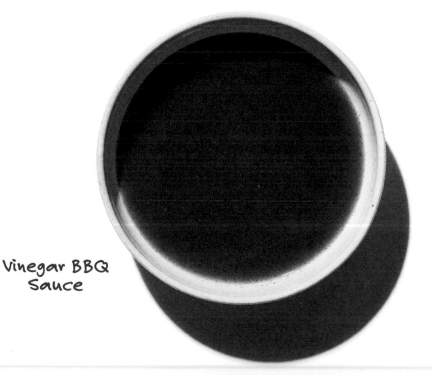

Vinegar BBQ
Sauce

Pit Mop

MAKES ABOUT 1½ GALLONS

A mop is basically a meat-moistening agent, and its main ingredient is vinegar. The mop also infuses a little flavor into the meat for an added layer of complexity. When pit cooking, we mop almost all of our long-cooking meats at varying intervals depending on how many pounds of meat we're dealing with. Each recipe has a specific time at which to open the pit and mop, ranging from every 15 minutes to every 30 after the meat's "crust" forms. Mopping is especially important in smoking because we're cooking with actual coals beneath the meat, and we don't want the meat to dry out. This technique can be useful whether you're cooking on a pit, a smoker, a grill, or even an oven.

INGREDIENTS

1 gallon distilled white vinegar

½ cup red pepper flakes

½ cup kosher salt

4 lemons, halved

1. Combine all the ingredients and ½ gallon of water in a large pot and set it over medium-high heat. Bring to a boil so that the pepper flakes open up and infuse the mop with flavor. Let the mop cool completely, about 1 hour.

2. Funnel the sauce into bottles or containers of your choice. Cover tightly. The sauce will keep, refrigerated, for up to 1 year. You can portion it out as you cook barbecue along the way.

How to Use a Mop

To apply the mop to the meat, take a brand-new floor mop, cut the handle to a size short enough so that it's easy to manipulate. Periodically use it to dab the liquid mop onto the meat to give it moisture. Alternatively, you can use any basting or cooking brush. The liquid mop helps the meat achieve that Southern-style barbecue flavor, which is what the mopping process is all about.

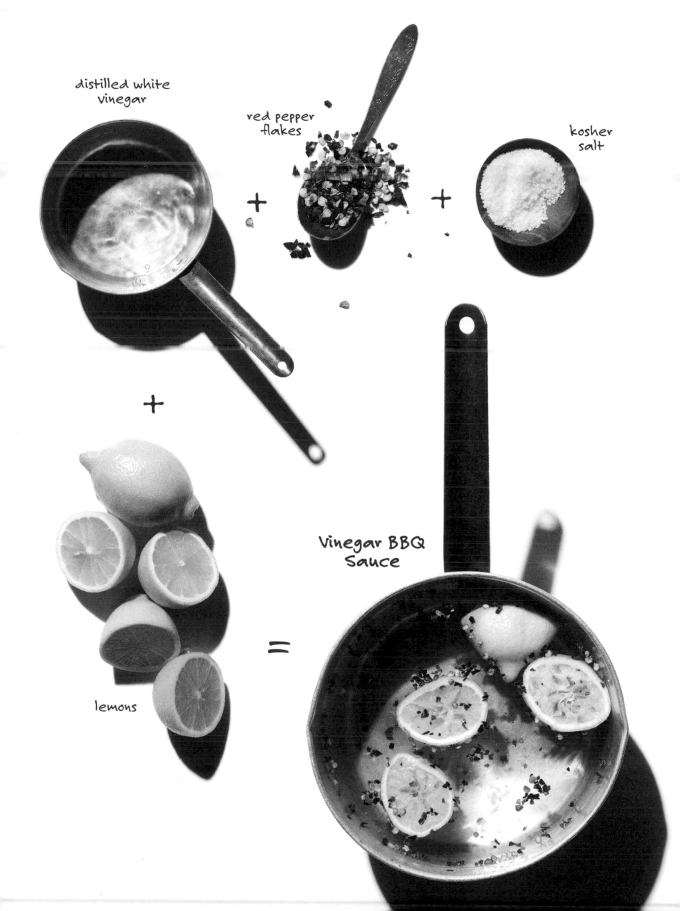

distilled white vinegar

+

red pepper flakes

+

kosher salt

+

lemons

=

Vinegar BBQ Sauce

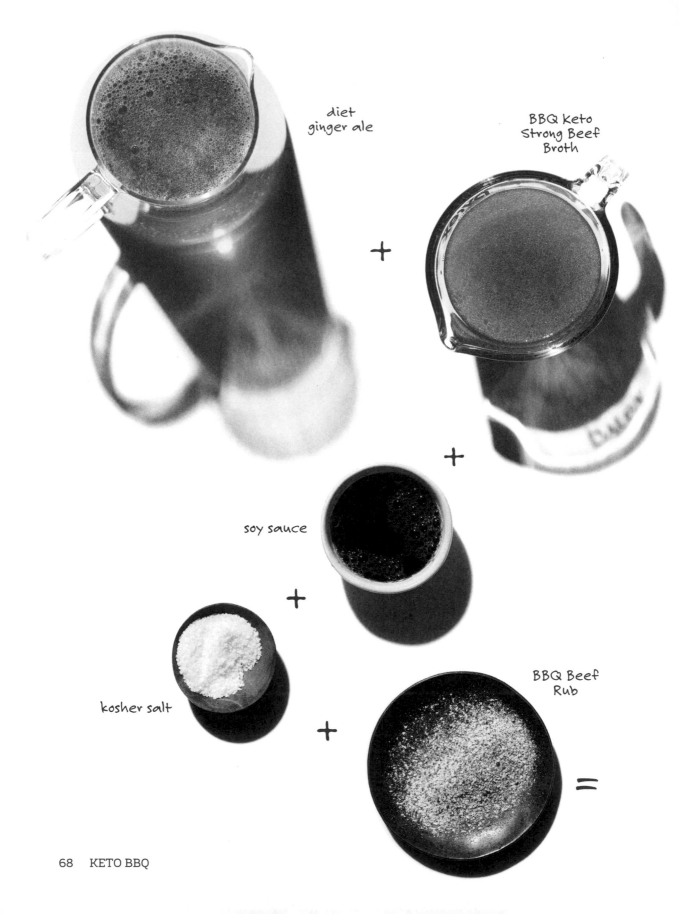

diet ginger ale

BBQ Keto Strong Beef Broth

+

+

soy sauce

+

kosher salt

+

BBQ Beef Rub

=

THE BASICS
Pit Marinade

Sometimes folks ask me if they can skip marinating meat. If I'm calling for you to marinate, it means you cannot skip this step. I don't do it unless it's necessary. Why is it sometimes important? Think about what a marinade does: Marinades are used to flavor and tenderize tougher cuts of meat. You soak meat in a marinade to help ensure that it won't dry out on the smoker. Brining works the same way, of course, but which process you use depends on what type and cut of meat you're cooking, how long you're cooking it, and over what kind of heat. Anything you soak in this marinade will be delicious.

INGREDIENTS

1 liter diet ginger ale

1 quart BBQ Keto Strong Beef Broth (*page 100*)

1½ cups soy sauce

2 cups kosher salt

¼ cup BBQ Beef Rub (*page 96*)

1. Combine all the ingredients in a large stock pot or similar container. Stir well to dissolve the salt and the rub thoroughly. Pour into a large bottle or other container, cover, and refrigerate for up to 2 weeks.

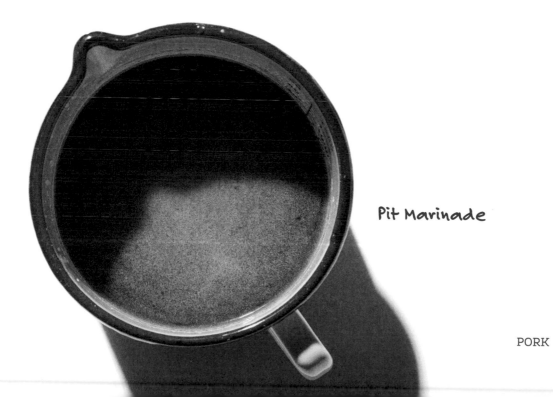

Pit Marinade

THE BASICS
Pit Spritz

MAKES 3 GENEROUS CUPS

People sometimes look at me funny when I reveal that the "secret" ingredient in my mouthwatering ribs is spritzing them with a solution that contains . . . liquid imitation butter. You know, the stuff that comes in a little bottle like vanilla extract in the supermarket baking aisle. For me, it offers an ingenious solve. Authentic melted butter is too thick to work in spray bottles, but the imitation butter works fine. This stuff does the trick of keeping your ribs moist during cooking. You can try spritzing other smoked meats with this solution, too.

INGREDIENTS

2 cups apple cider vinegar

1 cup white wine vinegar

1 tablespoon liquid imitation butter

1. In a large spray bottle, combine all the ingredients. Shake well to blend before using. If not using right away, pour the spritz into a large bottle or other container and refrigerate for up to 2 weeks.

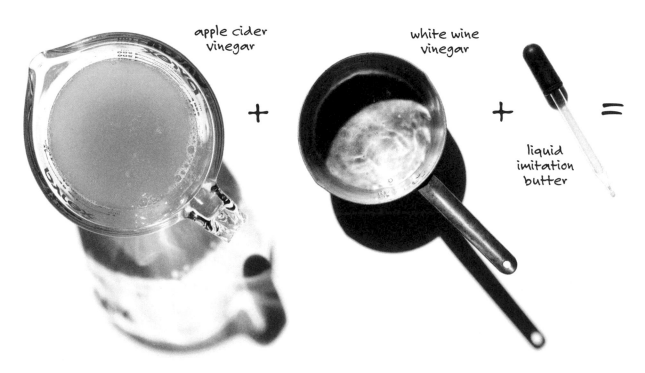

apple cider vinegar + white wine vinegar + liquid imitation butter =

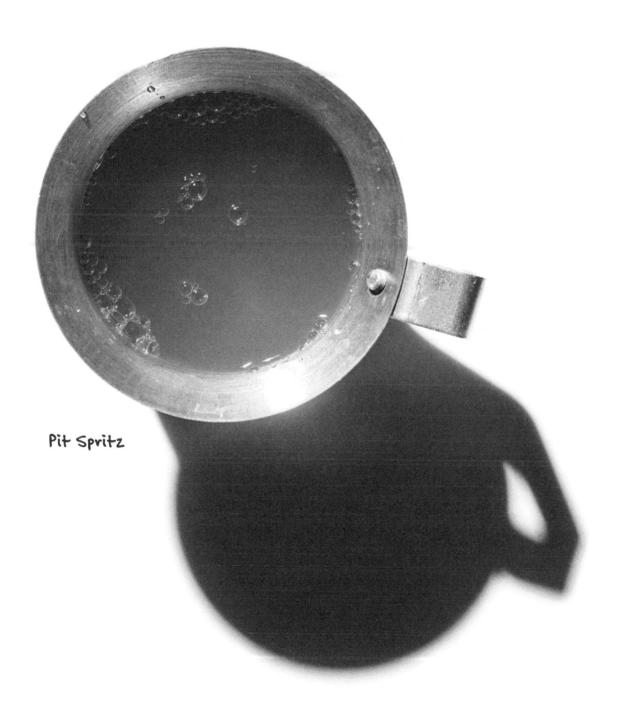

Pit Spritz

Smoked Pork Shoulder

A whole hog is not only my favorite thing in the world to cook, but it's also an absolute showstopper at any barbecue—from the annual World Barbecue Championships in Memphis to anything you might throw for friends and family in your backyard. There's nothing like the majesty of a whole hog that's just been laid out for your delectation. So why aren't I giving you a recipe for it? Look, I've given instructions on how to smoke whole hogs in my other books, and even I know that it's a special occasion food and a whole lot of work.

This book is about how to lead a BBQ Keto lifestyle on a day-in day-out basis. That's where the pork shoulder is your friend. And make no mistake about it: A whole bone-in pork shoulder is still somewhat of a project to cook. However, it is guaranteed not only to keep you on your diet plan but also to have plenty of delicious smoked meat to share with your family, friends, and neighbors, too.

To make this, you will need to prepare the Pit Mop recipe (page 66) and Vinegar BBQ Sauce (page 64), in advance.

INGREDIENTS

15- to 20-pound bone-in, whole pork shoulder

1 cup distilled white vinegar

Kosher salt and freshly ground black pepper

1½ gallons Pit Mop (*page 66*)

3½ cups Vinegar BBQ Sauce (*page 64*)

1. Select and prep the meat. My daddy didn't trim pork shoulders too much; maybe he cut away extra skin or large hunks of sinew hanging off a shoulder, but mostly he kept it simple and liked to take the shoulders straight from the butcher. Do it like he did: lay the shoulder out on a table covered with butcher paper or another sanitary covering, then rub it down all over the inside and the outside with white vinegar. Season all over with salt and pepper.

2. Heat your smoker to 250°F.

3. Place the shoulder in a large aluminum pan, meat-side down. Transfer the pan to the smoker and cook for 3 hours.

4. Remove the pan from the heat. Poke the skin with a sharp knife in three places. Using heat insulated gloves or tongs, carefully flip the shoulder so that it is now skin-side down. Cover the pan with aluminum foil.

5. Return the shoulder to the smoker. Cook for about 6 hours, all the while keeping the smoker temperature consistent at 250°F. Every hour, open up your smoker, remove the foil covering, and mop your meat.

6. After four hours, start checking the meat for doneness. My dad did this by grabbing the blade bone and pulling it. (Wear your heavy-duty work gloves to do this, if you like.) You want that meat to be almost falling-off-the-bone tender. If the bones are slipping easily, we're going to pull the shoulder out. If not, we're going on for 1 to 2 hours more. Again, we're mopping at 90-minute intervals until the meat is done. It's done when the temperature is 205°F.

7. When the meat is done: Pull it from the smoker and let it rest for 1 hour. My dad pulled all the meat from the shoulders by hand and with tongs, simply grabbing off pieces and collecting them in a large aluminum pan. At this point, we'd lightly sauce the meat with a vinegar-based sauce right there and make barbecue platters or sandwiches. For this recipe, use Vinegar BBQ Sauce. You'll notice you've got a lot of skin left over, which is perfect for making cracklings (see page 90)!

Smoked St. Louis Spareribs

Some of y'all might already know that spareribs are the long bones form the lower part of the hog's belly behind its shoulder—these are the least expensive ribs you can buy, and they are long, straight, and often fattier than baby backs. And by the way, they're often referred to as "St. Louis" because of the style of the cut: St. Louis ribs are just spareribs that have been squared off so they're uniform in size (or close to it). I'll tell you how to square off your spareribs, but you don't have to if you don't feel like it. A rack of spareribs usually weighs about 3 ½ pounds or less, which is why you might sometimes hear butchers or barbecue folks like me refer to them as "3½ and down" ribs. I like these because the fat surrounding the meat means there's a good opportunity for flavor. It's key to cook these right—by which I mean spritz them as written in the recipe—so they won't dry out. You want these suckers to be moist, tender, and full of smoky flavor.

INGREDIENTS

4 racks St. Louis spareribs, each weighing about 3½ pounds

9½ cups Pit Marinade (*page 68*)

1 cup BBQ Beef Rub (*page 96*)

3 cups Pit Spritz (*page 70*)

1 cup BBQ Keto Strong Beef Broth (*page 100*)

1 cup Tangy Sweet BBQ Sauce (*page 32*)

1. You might want to size up the ribs before proceeding with the recipe. See the note on page 78 about sizing the ribs.

2. Once they are sized (or not), trim the ribs. Place the slabs of ribs on a cutting board, bone-sides down. One by one, trim the excess fat from the first three ribs in the rack. If your butcher or grocer hasn't removed the thick weblike membrane ("the silver") that covers the bottom of the ribs, you need to do this. If you don't do this crucial step, the rub and other seasonings will not adhere to the meat. An easy way to do it is to make a small incision just below the length of the breastbone, and then work your fingers underneath the membrane until you have 2 or 3 inches cleared. Grab the membrane (sometimes it's easier to do this with a towel, as the membrane can be sticky), and gently but firmly pull the membrane away from the ribs. Once you've done this, discard the silver and use a sharp paring knife to trim any additional fat from the racks.

3. After the ribs are properly trimmed, set the racks in an aluminum baking pan, large enough so that they can all fit flat (or use 2 pans and divide the ribs). Pour the marinade over the ribs to cover them completely. Cover the pan with aluminum foil and let the ribs rest, refrigerated, for 4 hours.

4. When you are ready to cook the ribs, remove them from the marinade and discard the marinade. Rinse the ribs in cold water and thoroughly pat them dry with paper towels or a clean kitchen towel. Apply the rub lightly around the edges of the ribs, over the back side of them, and on top. Let the ribs rest, lightly tented with foil, at room temperature for 30 minutes while you prepare your smoker.

5. Heat your smoker to 275°F.

6. Transfer the ribs to a large clean baking pan or two small ones. Put the ribs in the smoker and cook for 3 hours, taking care to keep your heat consistent. After the first 45 minutes of cooking time, open the smoker and hit the ribs with the spritz. Continue to spritz the ribs every 15 minutes after that, for the duration of the 3 hours.

7. After 3 hours of smoking and spritzing, remove the pan from the smoker. Pour the broth into a clean and deep aluminum baking pan. Place the ribs in the pan, bone-side down, and cover the pan with foil. Place the pan in the smoker for 2 hours longer.

8. After 2 hours, remove the pan from the smoker and shut off the heat. Remove the foil cover and use a brush to glaze the ribs lightly and all over with the Tangy Sweet BBQ Sauce. Cover the pan with foil, return it to the smoker, and let the ribs rest in the smoker for 1 hour as the smoker's temperature gradually decreases.

9. After 1 hour, remove the ribs from the pan and transfer them to a cutting board. Let them rest 10 additional minutes, and then cut and serve.

Blackberry Spareribs

MAKES 3 RACKS, SERVES 4 TO 6

Blackberries happen to be my favorite fruit. When I started on the Keto lifestyle, one of the easiest things for me to do was replace the processed junk food snacks I was eating with pints of blackberries. I just carry them around with me everywhere I go. That's what inspired me to try to figure out a recipe that would combine ribs with the distinct sweet-tart flavor of blackberries. My next challenge was how to prepare the ribs without any added sugar so I could enjoy sweet ribs while still keeping my body within the guidelines of the Keto plan. Here's what I came up with: Ribs that are literally finger-lickin' good!

INGREDIENTS

RIBS:

3 racks St. Louis spareribs, each weighing about 2½ to 3 pounds

1 cup vegetable oil

1 cup BBQ Beef Rub (*page 96*)

SPRITZ:

2 cups BBQ Keto Strong Beef Broth (*page 100*)

1-ounce bottle McCormick Imitation Butter Extract

2 tablespoons monk fruit sweetener (*see page 19*)

BLACKBERRY SAUCE:

1 cup Tangy Sweet BBQ Sauce (*page 32*)

1 tablespoon monk fruit sweetener

2 cups sugar-free blackberry jam

FOR THE RIBS:

1. Remove the membrane from the back of the ribs and trim the excess fat. Apply a light coating of oil to the ribs and then a coat of rub on top. Transfer the ribs to an aluminum baking pan.

2. Preheat the smoker or oven to 275°F.

3. Place the ribs in the smoker for 3 hours.

FOR THE SPRITZ:

1. Mix all the ingredients for the spritz in a small pot set over medium heat. Heat just until the monk fruit sweetener is dissolved. Remove from the stove, set aside to cool, and then transfer to a spray bottle.

2. Once the ribs have been in the smoker for 1 hour, spritz them every 15 minutes for the next hour. After the second hour, wrap the pan holding the ribs in foil and finish cooking until the internal temperature of the meat between the bones of the ribs is 205°F.

FOR THE BLACKBERRY SAUCE:

1. Put all the ingredients in a blender and puree until smooth.

2. When the ribs reach 205°F, unwrap the foil and apply the blackberry sauce on the top and bottom of the ribs. Return the pan to the smoker for 10 minutes for the sauce to set.

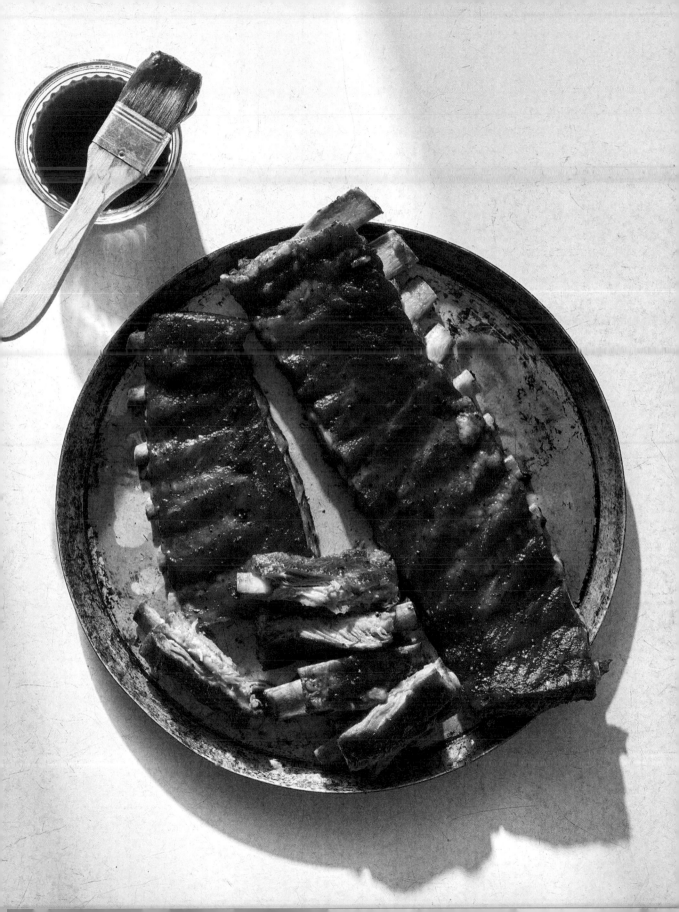

How to Size Up the Ribs

You can "size up" your ribs as we do in competition, which just means to ensure that they're all about the same length. This is much easier to do with spareribs than with baby backs because sparerib bones are straight and flat and not curved.

Sizing up the ribs improves their appearance and is good for ensuring a consistent cooking time, too—but you don't have to do it. If you do, it takes two cuts. Use a sharp boning knife to first remove the flap of meat at the end of the rack. To do this, look at the narrower end of the rack and locate the last, shortest bone. There's usually a portion of meat attached to that bone that's loose. To remove it, make a vertical cut parallel to, and about ½ inch away from, that last bone. Next, make a horizontal cut to separate the bone and cartilage.

To find the sweet spot, first find the longest rib, usually the fourth bone in on the wider end of the rack. Feel along that rib until you detect a softer spot, which is a cartilaginous section where the rib connects to the breastbone. All the other ribs connect to the breastbone in the same way. Make the cut by inserting the knife into the soft spot, and then slicing perpendicular to the ribs, cutting through all the soft spots where each rib meets the breastbone. Once the breastbone is removed, you will have a clean rectangular rack of ribs, easy to cook and just about perfect for eating. The finished rack should end up about 5 to 6 inches long.

Competition Baby Back Ribs

MAKES 4 RACKS, SERVES 4 TO 6

I wish I had a nickel for every time someone has come up to me at a barbecue contest to tell me that baby back ribs are their number-one favorite food. Guess what? Baby backs are among my favorite foods, too.

I don't mind telling you that I like spareribs, plenty, too. But I like baby backs the best. These are the ribs that separate the loin section from the tenderloin. They're small and cute and seem to require less work to hold and eat. Which is why so many people love them. In barbecue cooking competitions, my ribs have been the linchpins to my success. You simply cannot become Grand Champion at Memphis in May, the World Championship barbecue cooking contest, without mastering baby back ribs. And what those judges look for in a winning rib is that ideal combination of texture (soft meat, yet it can't be mushy), smoky flavor (but with a little sweetness to it), and a shiny, appealing appearance on the plate.

Here's how I get that perfect balance of natural sweetness.

INGREDIENTS

4 racks baby back ribs, each weighing about 3 pounds

3 cups Pit Marinade (*page 68*)

2 cups BBQ Keto Rub (*page 96*)

3 cups Pit Spritz (*page 70*)

1 cup BBQ Keto Strong Beef Broth (*page 100*)

2 cups Hickory BBQ Sauce (*page 99*)

1. One at a time, place the racks on a cutting board, bone-side up. If your butcher or grocer hasn't removed the thick weblike membrane ("the silver") that covers the ribs, you'll need to do it. If you don't do this crucial step, the rub and other seasonings will not adhere to the meat. An easy way to remove the silver is to make a small incision just below the length of the breastbone, and then work your fingers underneath the membrane until you have 2 or 3 inches cleared. Grab the membrane (sometimes it's easier to do that with a towel, as this can be sticky), and gently but firmly pull the membrane away from the ribs. Once you've done this, discard the silver and use a sharp paring knife to trim any additional fat from the racks.

recipe continues

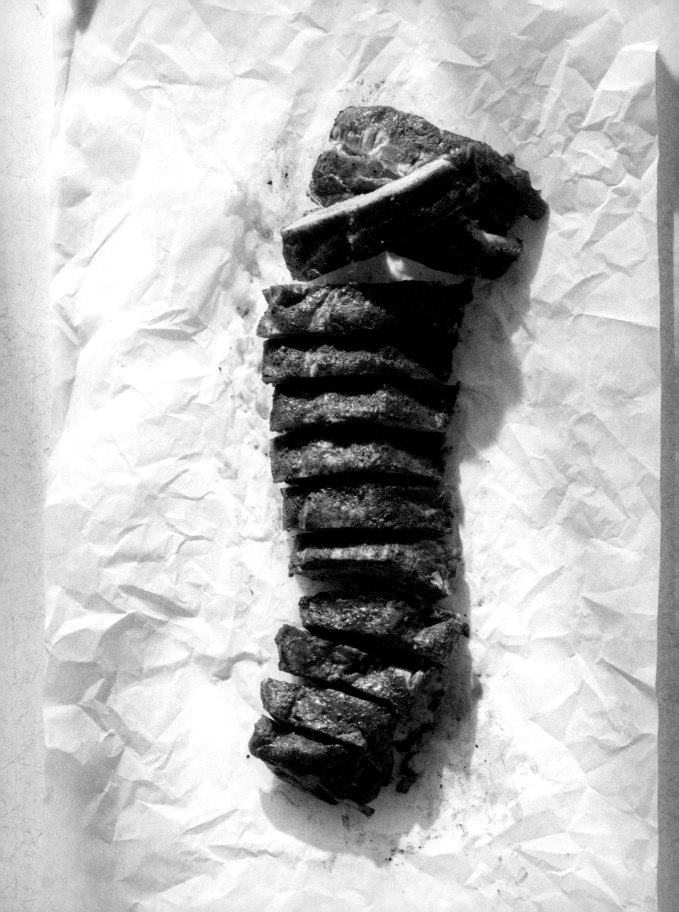

2. After the ribs are properly trimmed, set the racks in a large aluminum baking pan big enough to allow them to fit in a single layer (or use 2 pans and divide the ribs). Pour the marinade over the ribs to cover completely. Cover the pan with aluminum foil and put in refrigerator for 1 hour.

3. When you are ready to cook the ribs, remove them from the marinade and discard the marinade. Pat the ribs dry all over with paper towels or a clean kitchen towel. Apply the BBQ Keto Rub lightly around the edges of the ribs, over the back sides of them, and on top. Then let the ribs rest, lightly tented with foil, at room temperature for 30 minutes while you prepare your smoker.

4. Heat the smoker to 250°F.

5. Transfer the ribs to a clean baking pan, put it in the smoker, and cook for 2 hours, taking care to keep the heat consistent. After the first 45 minutes of cooking time, open the smoker and hit the ribs with the spritz. Continue to spritz the ribs every 15 minutes after that until the ribs have been on the smoker for 3 hours.

6. Remove the pan from the smoker. Pour the broth into a clean, deep baking pan. Transfer the ribs to the new pan, bone-sides down, and cover the pan with foil. Place the pan back in the smoker and continue to smoke for 1 hour.

7. After 1 hour, remove the pan from the smoker and shut off the heat on the smoker. Remove the foil and use a brush to glaze the ribs lightly and all over with the Hickory BBQ Sauce. Re-cover the pan, return it to the smoker, and let the ribs rest in the smoker for 30 minutes.

8. After 30 minutes, remove the pan from the smoker and transfer the ribs to a cutting board. Let them rest for 10 additional minutes, and then cut between the bones and serve.

Smoked Pork Belly Bites

SERVES 6

Pork belly sliders are everywhere now. When I was growing up, "pork belly" just meant a particularly inexpensive, fatty cut of meat from the underside of a hog's belly near its loin. Yes, I'm well aware that when the skin is removed from this belly and is then salted and cured, it's bacon. I am also aware that it's very easy to make something delicious out of this trendy ingredient, and to make it in a Keto-friendly way. This is a tempting treat for a backyard barbecue—great to snack on with your cocktails (see page 171).

INGREDIENTS

3- to 3½-pound section of pork belly

¾ cup BBQ Beef Rub (*page 96***)**

½ cup Tangy Sweet BBQ Sauce (*page 32***)**

1. If the pork belly still has its skin (or "rind") on it, use a sharp knife to remove as much of it as possible, but don't lose too much of the fat.

2. Use a sharp knife to cube the belly into bite-size nuggets, about 1½ inches square. Apply the rub all over the pork belly bites, covering the tops, bottoms, and sides. Use your fingers to rub it into the meat and transfer the covered bites to a medium-sized aluminum pan.

3. Heat the smoker to 225°F.

4. Place the pan on the smoker and cook the belly bites until the internal temperature of one of the fattest bites reaches 165°F, about 3½ hours.

5. Remove the pan from the smoker. Toss the bites with Tangy Sweet BBQ Sauce to coat. Return the pan to the smoker for 10 additional minutes for the sauce to set.

6. Remove the bites from the smoker. Enjoy as appetizers with your cocktails or serve with a side of Mama's Classic Slaw (*page 130*) for dinner, if you like.

Grilled "Honey" Mustard Pork Chops

SERVES 4

It's always a good rule of thumb to brine pork chops before grilling. Because pork chops are fairly lean, submerging them in a brine does two things. First, it keeps the meat moist by introducing extra moisture, which provides a little insurance in case the meat gets a little overcooked. Second, it evenly seasons the meat beyond the surface only.

INGREDIENTS

6 cups cold water

⅓ cup kosher salt

1 tablespoon monk fruit sweetener (*see page 19*)

4 garlic cloves, smashed

1 teaspoon freshly ground black pepper

4 thick bone-in pork rib chops (each weighing 12 to 16 ounces and at least 1 inch thick)

½ cup BBQ Beef Rub (*page 96*)

1 cup Keto "Honey" Mustard Sauce (*page 162*)

1. To brine the pork chops, pour the water into a large bowl. Add the salt, monk fruit sweetener, garlic cloves, and pepper and whisk constantly until the sugar and salt dissolve and incorporate. Submerge the pork chops in the brine, cover the bowl, and refrigerate for at least 30 minutes or up to 2 hours.

2. About 20 minutes before you're ready to cook, heat an outdoor grill. For a charcoal grill, arrange lit coals on one side of the grill, and leave the other half empty. For a gas grill, heat the burners to high (at least 450°F).

3. When you are ready to cook, lift the chops from the brine and use paper towels or a clean kitchen towel to pat them dry all over. Season the pork chops all over with BBQ Beef Rub. If using a charcoal grill, place all of the pork chops on the rack above the hotter side of the grill. If using a gas grill, lower one of the burners to medium heat and transfer the chops onto the racks. Grill for 3 minutes, or until grill marks appear on the bottom of the pork chops.

recipe continues

4. If using a charcoal grill, when you've got good grill marks on the bottom of your pork chops, transfer them to the cooler part of the grill. Cover both of the grills and continue to cook the pork chops, checking them every 2 minutes, until the thickest piece registers 145°F on an instant-read thermometer. (Go a few minutes more if you want them to be well-done, but remember that the internal temperature will increase as the meat rests.)

5. When the pork chops are done, transfer them to a cutting board or serving platter. Tent them loosely with aluminum foil and allow them to rest for 10 minutes. Serve each pork chop with ¼ cup of the Keto "Honey" Mustard Sauce poured over it.

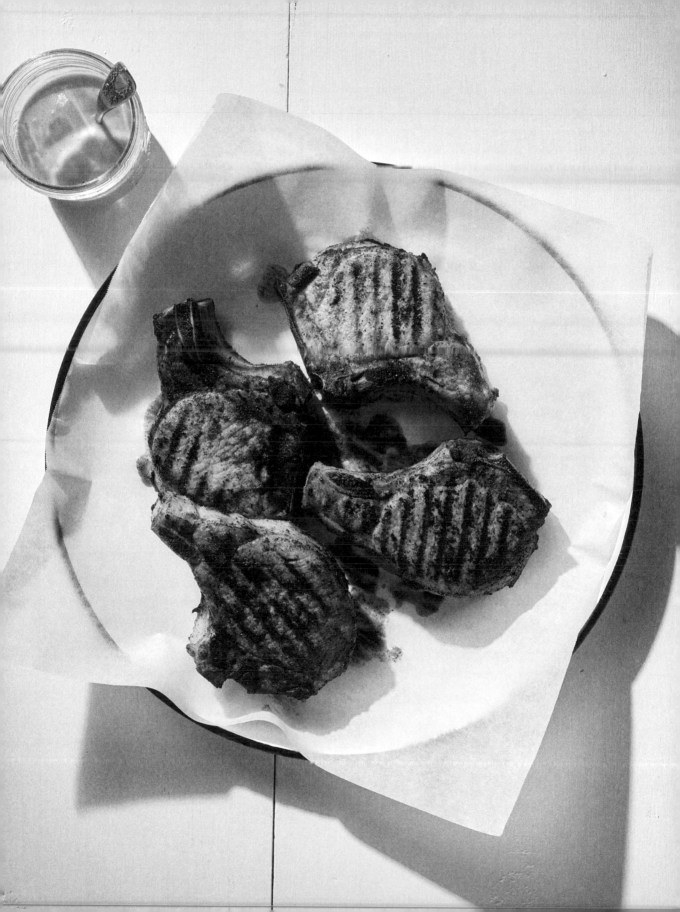

Roasted Apple and Sausage-Stuffed Pork Chops

SERVES 4

This dish is how I answer the question of what I eat on nights when I don't fire up my smoker. Yes, folks, sometimes I do actually use an oven—it might be raining outside, you never know. I like pork chops because they're a great piece of meat to sink your teeth into, and they don't have a whole lot of natural fat on them. This means that pork chops generally need a little help in the flavor department. Here's how I do it. This'll be the best pork chop you ever had. Well, maybe the best one that ever came out of your oven instead of your smoker.

INGREDIENTS

4 thick bone-in pork rib chops (weighing 12 to 16 ounces each and at least 1½ inches thick)

4 cups unsweetened coconut milk

1 cup distilled white vinegar

1 pound ground fresh pork sausage, removed from casing

1 apple, peeled and finely diced

1 cup BBQ Beef Rub (*page 96*)

1 pound green beans, trimmed

1 red bell pepper, seeds removed and pepper thinly sliced

1 medium white onion, thinly sliced

2 tablespoons hickory smoked salt (you can substitute pink Himalayan salt or kosher salt)

2 cups Tangy Sweet BBQ Sauce (*page 32*)

1. Place the pork chops in a large plastic bag and pour in the coconut milk and vinegar. Seal tightly and refrigerate for at least 4 hours or overnight.

2. Preheat the oven to 375°F.

3. When you are ready to cook the pork chops, combine the sausage and diced apple in a medium bowl and use your hands to mix them together. Lift the pork chops from the marinade and discard the marinade. Use a sharp paring knife to cut a 2-inch-long slit about 2 inches deep in the side opposite the bone of each chop. This will make a pocket. Stuff the sausage mixture deep into the pocket of each pork chop. For each pork chop, use three toothpicks to close the pocket and hold the sausage mixture in place. Season both sides of each chop with the rub.

4. Put the green beans, red pepper strips, and sliced onions in the bottom of a 13-by-9-inch baking dish. Arrange the pork chops in a single layer on top. Sprinkle the chops with the smoked salt or any salt you're using.

5. Place the pan in the oven and cook for 30 minutes. Remove the pan from the oven, flip the pork chops, and brush them with the Tangy Sweet BBQ Sauce. Cook for an additional 20 minutes, or until a thermometer inserted into the thickest part of the chop reads 145°F.

6. Remove the pan from the oven. Transfer the chops to a platter or plate and let rest, loosely covered with foil, for 10 minutes. Serve them up with the green beans, peppers and onions.

Backyard Pork Loins

SERVES 8 TO 10

There's probably no bigger bang for your buck when it comes to pleasing your dinner guests than pork loin—it looks like a fancy roast, yet it's a very simple thing to prepare. I like it because it's easy to smoke, feeds a lot of folks, is next to impossible to mess up, and is not as time consuming as a pork shoulder. This is your go-to for a casual barbecue with friends and family.

INGREDIENTS

6 cups cold water

⅓ cup kosher salt

1 tablespoon monk fruit sweetener (*see page 19*)

4 cloves garlic, peeled and smashed

1 teaspoon black pepper

2 3½- to 4-pound boneless pork loin roasts

2 cups BBQ Beef Rub (*page 96*)

2 cups Tangy Sweet BBQ Sauce (*page 32*)

1. Pour the cold water into a large bowl or pot. Add the salt, monk fruit sweetener, garlic cloves, and pepper and whisk until the sweetener and salt dissolve. Submerge the loins in the brine, cover the bowl, and refrigerate for up to 4 hours.

2. When you are ready to cook the pork loins, heat the smoker to 350°F.

3. Remove the bowl from the refrigerator. Discard the brine and transfer the pork loins to a cutting board. Pat the pork loins dry and use your fingers to apply the rub all over them. Put the loins in a medium aluminum baking pan in the smoker and cook for 1½ hours or until the middle of each loin registers 155°F on an instant-read thermometer.

4. Remove the pan from the smoker and use a brush to apply the sauce all over both loins. Return the pan to the smoker and cook the loins for an additional 15 minutes.

5. Remove the pan from the smoker and let the loins rest, loosely covered with foil, for 30 minutes. Slice the loins into ½-inch-thick slices and serve.

Chorizo-Stuffed Pork Tenderloin

SERVES 4

Just because pork tenderloins are thin and small doesn't mean they can't benefit from that world-famous Georgia smoked meat cooking process. Yes, this is a lean and tender piece of meat that comes from the muscle that runs along a hog's backbone (unlike the loin, which, though it sounds like it would be similar, is much wider and fattier). Tenderloin is lean and dries out easily, so I like stuffing it with this chorizo, which adds a lot of fat and a lot of flavor.

INGREDIENTS

1 large pork tenderloin (weighing about 2 pounds)

1 pound chorizo sausage links

½ cup BBQ Beef Rub (*page 96*)

1 cup Vinegar BBQ Sauce (*page 64*)

1. Heat the smoker to 300°F.

2. Use paper towels or a clean kitchen towel to pat the tenderloin dry all over. Insert a sharp paring or boning knife with a long, thin, straight blade through the center of the tenderloin. Take care not to cut out to the sides but instead insert the knife about 1 inch into the center. Remove the knife and then slowly and firmly push the plastic tube of a turkey baster through the cut to enlarge the opening all the way through the tenderloin.

3. Trim the sausage links to the length of the tenderloin. Stuff it into the opening and use your fingers to apply the rub all over the tenderloin, coating it well on the outside. Place the tenderloin in a medium-sized aluminum pan and transfer the pan to the smoker. Cook the tenderloin for about 1 hour or until the middle of the loin registers 150°F on an instant-read thermometer.

4. During the last 15 minutes of cooking time, use half the Vinegar BBQ Sauce and a brush to glaze the tenderloin. Reserve the remaining sauce.

5. Remove the pan from the smoker. Allow the meat to rest, loosely tented with foil, for 10 minutes. Cut the loins into slices about ½ inch thick and serve drizzled with the sauce.

Pork Cracklings

Pork cracklings is what I grew up calling fried pig skins—same as pork rinds, just by a different name. Pork rinds are a godsend for folks following the Keto plan because they're full of fat and flavor and have zero carbs or sugars. I use them crumbled up and in place of breadcrumbs (see Southern "Fried" Chicken Tenders, page 46). I have seen folks use them as a base for nachos instead of tortilla chips. I can tell you that they're cheap to buy in stores but more delicious when you make your own. Here's a way to do so without having to deep fry them.

INGREDIENTS

2 pounds pork rind with about 1 inch of fat

2 tablespoons fine sea salt

1. Preheat the oven to 400°F.

2. Clean the rind by washing it in cold water and using paper towels or a clean kitchen towel to dry it thoroughly.

3. Use a very sharp knife or kitchen shears to cut the rind into 1-inch squares.

4. Find a baking pan fitted with a rack and arrange the squares in a single layer on the rack so that they are sitting about ½ inch or so above the pan. Sprinkle the strips with 1 tablespoon of the salt.

5. Bake the strips for 10 minutes, flip them, and continue cooking for 10 minutes more or until they are puffed, golden, and crisp. There will be bubbles on their surface. Remove from the oven and sprinkle with the remaining tablespoon of salt. Allow the rinds to cool completely.

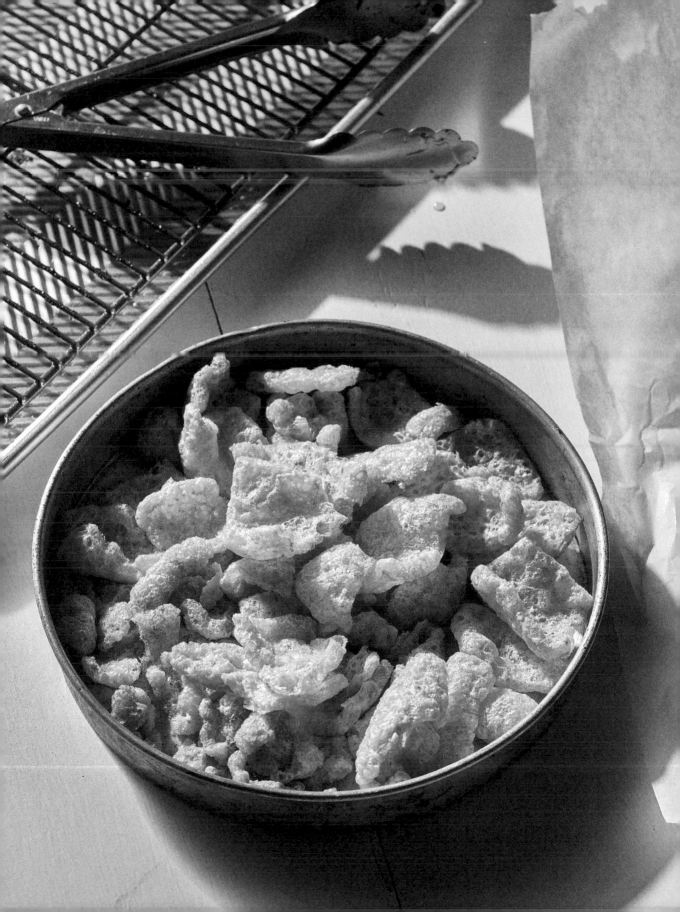

CHAPTER 4

Beef

I SURE HOPE I DON'T HAVE TO EXPLAIN TO ANYONE HOW DELICIOUS BEEF IS. I also hope that I don't have to tell anyone interested in the Keto lifestyle that eating beef is a good idea. Most cuts have lots of fat, and consuming fat is a big part of what makes following the Keto diet such a successful way to lose weight and keep it off. What a lot of folks assume, though, is that people on Keto eating plans do nothing but shove burgers—without the bun, of course—into their pieholes. The fact is, once you do a little research on Keto you learn that all fats are not created equal, and that some are much better for you than others (and some, like saturated fats, are downright bad for you).

So, where does beef fall? Well, beef contains equal amounts of monounsaturated fats, the so-called "good fats" (the same ones in olive oil and avocados) which are good for you, and saturated fats. People used to think that saturated fats were terrible for you, but more recent studies have shown that saturated fats can actually increase the so-called "heart healthy" HDL "good" cholesterol. Together, the fats in meats help decrease the risk of heart attacks and stroke and are not only okay but good to eat. But as with everything else on the Keto diet, you can never just go hog wild with anything. The eating plan is about balance, so you want to make sure you're getting plenty of the "good fats" from items that are not meat or dairy, such as nuts, seeds, and oily fish such as salmon. Why am I pausing to give you this brief lecture on fat when I am just about to give you a glorious and mouthwatering collection of beef recipes? Balance is the keyword. Be sure a big hunk o' steak is not the only thing on your plate. We all want to stay healthy and eat balanced meals, so turn to the Vegetables and Greens chapter (*page 125*) when you are doing your meal planning.

Now, how about that big hunk o' steak? Yeah, I got you covered. I got the best burger you'll ever inhale, too. And I've got more than that for you in this chapter. On the competitive barbecue circuit hog, of course, dominates the proceedings. But I'll let y'all in on a little-known fact. Beef is my secret weapon at barbecue contests. That's because if you're good at cooking a brisket, you can win a whole lot of prize money and make yourself stand out from the folks who only know how to cook hogs. Because brisket is a big, dense, tough cut of beef from a steer's shoulder, some folks just don't want to fool with it or learn what it takes to get it right. But getting good at smoking brisket has been my ticket to a lot of winners' podiums. And let me assure you that once you learn how to be patient and methodical when smoking brisket, you'll get it right every time. It will be that perfect combination of chewy and tender with that gorgeous pink smoke ring around the meat. Even better than that, folks, is looking nice and slim and trim when you're eating it because you're on Keto.

RECIPES

THE BASICS:

THE BASICS
BBQ Beef Rub

MAKES ABOUT 2 CUPS

Cuts of beef that are rich and fatty have their own distinctive flavor and character, and your job as the backyard pitmaster is to figure out how to create seasoning combinations that work with that flavor rather than overwhelming it. When I created my beef rub, I was looking to combine some strong, savory flavors that could hold their own with the beef and with each other. Adding the monk fruit sweetener means we get rid of the sugar I used to include in my beef rubs, but we still keep a hint of natural sweetness.

INGREDIENTS

1 cup kosher salt

⅓ cup black pepper

1 teaspoon monk fruit sweetener (*see page 19*)

1 teaspoon chipotle powder

1 teaspoon mild, medium, or hot chili powder

1 tablespoon garlic powder

1 tablespoon granulated dried onion

1. In a large bowl, combine all the ingredients and stir until well mixed. Store the rub in an airtight container, away from heat and light, for up to 6 months.

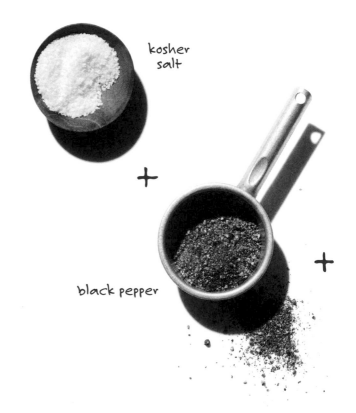

kosher salt

black pepper

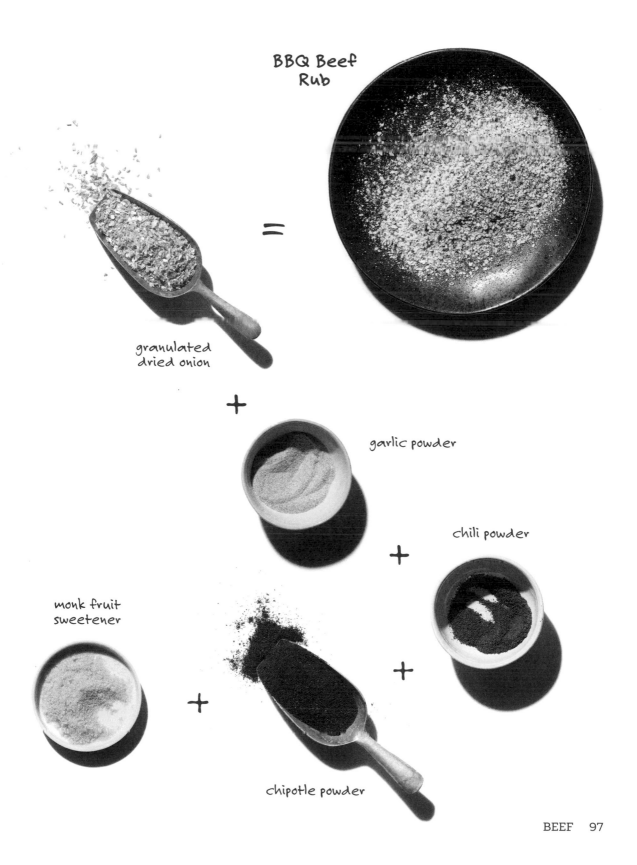

BBQ Beef
Rub

granulated
dried onion

=

+

garlic powder

chili powder

+

monk fruit
sweetener

+

chipotle powder

+

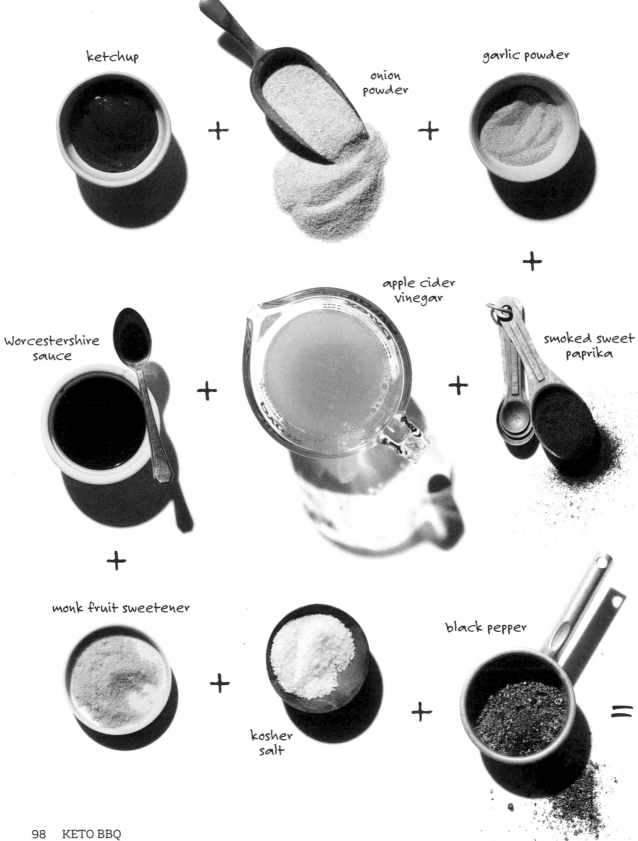

ketchup + onion powder + garlic powder + Worcestershire sauce + apple cider vinegar + smoked sweet paprika + monk fruit sweetener + kosher salt + black pepper =

Hickory BBQ Sauce

MAKES ABOUT 3½ CUPS

I've tasted too many batches of perfectly good barbecue sauce ruined by being too sweet. Beef has a natural sweetness to it, so you don't want to make it even sweeter. This sauce does just the opposite and will never be too sweet for brisket, beef ribs, or burgers. In particular, the paprika in the sauce adds depth and enhances the smoky flavor of what's naturally going on in the smoker.

INGREDIENTS

2 cups ketchup

2 tablespoons onion powder

2 tablespoons garlic powder

2 tablespoons smoked sweet paprika

⅔ cup apple cider vinegar

2 tablespoons Worcestershire sauce

2 tablespoons monk fruit sweetener (*see page 19*)

2 tablespoons kosher salt

2 tablespoons black pepper

1. In the canister of a large blender, combine all the ingredients. Pulse until thoroughly combined. Pour the sauce into a saucepan and set it over medium heat. Stirring continuously, let the sauce heat through but do not allow it to boil. When the ingredients are thoroughly combined, remove the pan from the heat. Use the sauce warm, if you like, or let it cool to room temperature. If reserving for a later use, allow the mixture to cool and then pour it into a large bottle or other container. Tightly cover and refrigerate for up to 6 months. Warm before using, if you like.

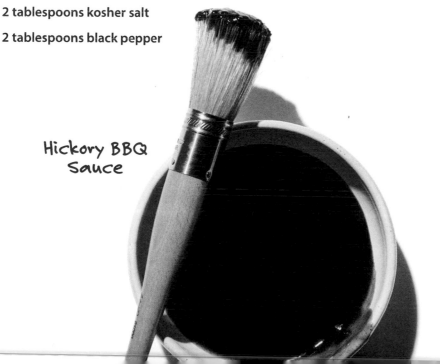

Hickory BBQ Sauce

THE BASICS
BBQ Keto Strong Beef Broth

MAKES 6 TO 8 CUPS

This full-flavored broth calls for oxtail bones, but you can use a combination of oxtail bones, chicken bones, chicken feet, marrow bones, or whatever you've got handy. The best tip for making beef broth is to save the leftover bones from your favorite bone-in ribeye and use them to make some good clear, golden broth. And if you're roasting an entire chicken, save that carcass and use those bones, too. You can make this flavorful broth in a slow cooker, pressure cooker, or Dutch oven. It's great as a marinade or as a base for soups and sauces.

INGREDIENTS

4 pounds oxtail bones or other bones (*see headnote*)

10 cups water

1 medium white onion, halved and peeled

5 cloves garlic

1 tablespoon kosher salt

2 tablespoons peppercorns

2 tablespoons apple cider vinegar

3 fresh or dried bay leaves

1 tablespoon turmeric

1. Preheat the oven to 400°F.

2. Spread the bones on a lightly oiled sheet pan and sprinkle them with salt. Roast the bones until they are golden and crunchy, about 45 minutes.

3. Transfer the bones to the bowl of a pressure cooker, slow cooker, or Dutch oven. Top them with the water and add the onion, garlic, salt, peppercorns, vinegar, and bay leaves.

FOR A PRESSURE COOKER: Lock the lid of the pressure cooker and turn to high heat. Once it reaches high pressure according to the indicator, or you see a small amount of vapor escaping through the valve, turn to the lowest setting and let the broth cook for 90 minutes. When done, let the pressure release naturally for 15 minutes.

FOR A SLOW COOKER: Cover the cooker with the lid and cook for at least 6 hours on high or for up to 10 hours on low.

FOR A DUTCH OVEN: Place the pot over medium heat and bring to a rapid simmer. Reduce the heat to low so that the stock is at a very low simmer, with just a few bubbles breaking the surface. Cover and cook for about 6 hours, maintaining the heat at a low level so the stock does not boil dry. Watch the water level and add more if needed.

4. The stock is done when it is a rich, golden brown color. The texture should be slightly thick and even a little gelatinous rather than thin and watery. Remove the stock from the heat and let it rest for 15 minutes. Place a fine mesh sieve or strainer over a large bowl and carefully strain the broth into the bowl. Discard the bones and other ingredients, such as the peppercorns and bay leaves, and strain again. For very clear, golden broth, strain the stock two or three additional times to your desired clarity. Add the turmeric and stir until it dissolves.

5. Use the broth immediately or store it in sealed jars, refrigerated, for up to 5 days. Note that once the broth is chilled, it may become gelatinous and solid. This is because it is high in fat, in accordance with Keto principles. It will liquefy again once heated.

6. You can pour the stock into a freezer-safe container or large plastic bag, close tightly, and freeze for up to 6 months. Defrost the stock in the refrigerator for about 24 hours. For a quicker defrost, submerge the container in a bowl of cold water.

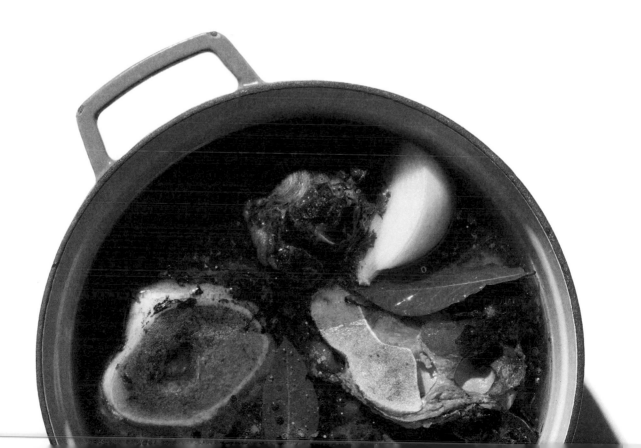

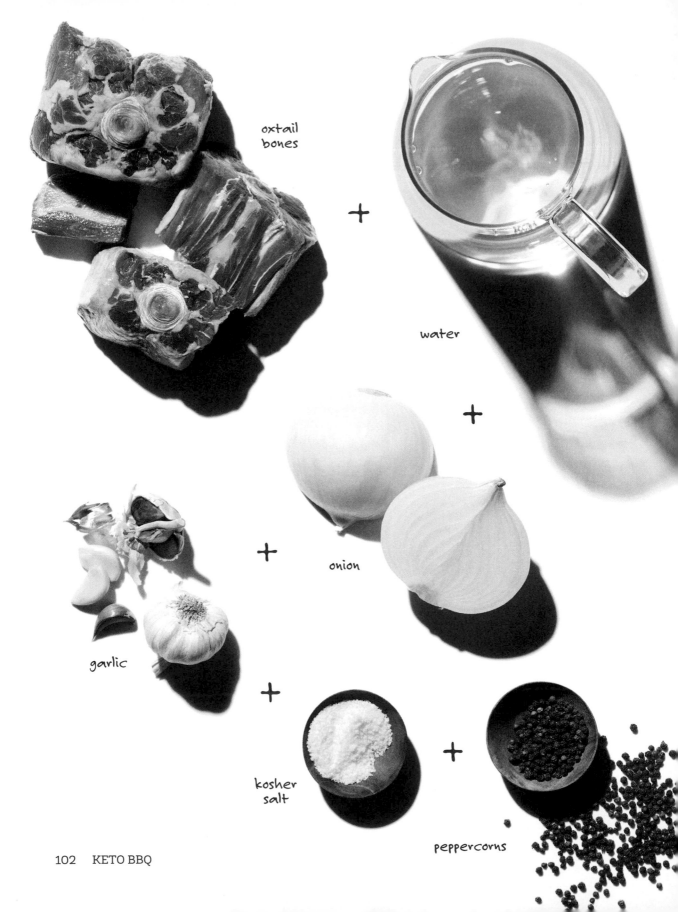

oxtail
bones

+

water

+

+

garlic

onion

+

kosher
salt

+

peppercorns

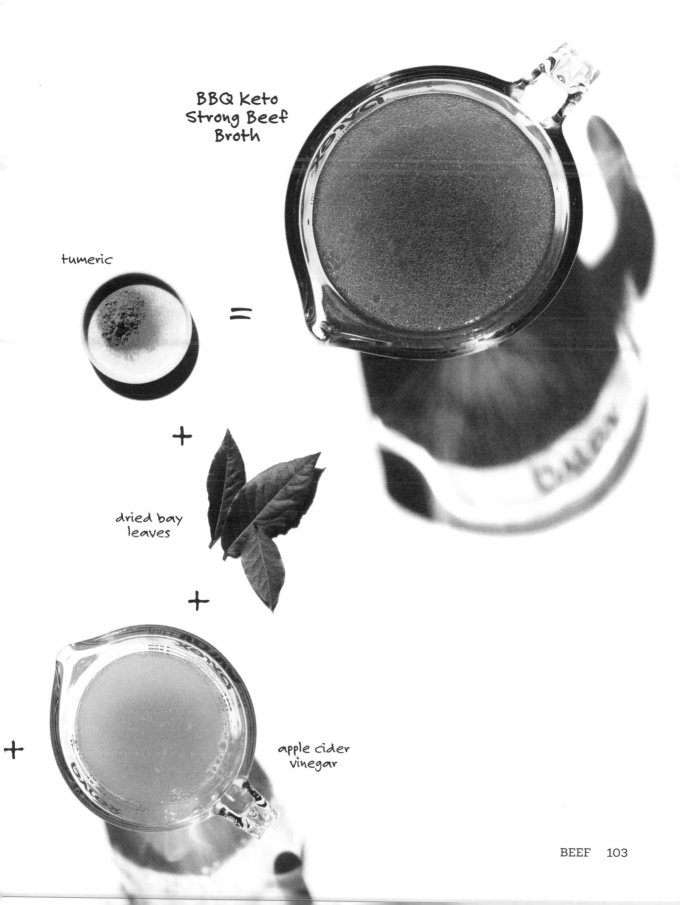

BBQ keto
Strong Beef
Broth

tumeric

=

+

dried bay
leaves

+

+

apple cider
vinegar

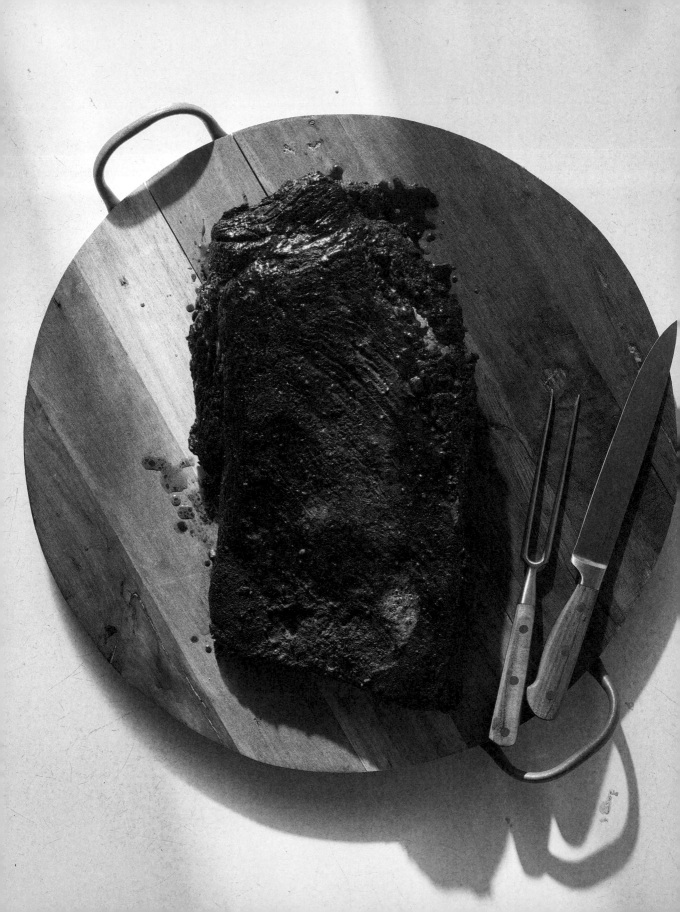

Prize-Winning Brisket & Burnt Ends

Hog folks like me just scratch our heads when we first encounter a brisket. I know I did. If you're from South Georgia, you didn't grow up with this on your table. We all eat what we have around us and what local customs dictate—and what we can afford, too. While it's a bit expensive now, brisket was traditionally a very inexpensive cut because it's so sinewy and tough. I won't pretend that I didn't have to try—*hard*—to figure out how to make this taste good. Many a weekend I was sweating it out in my backyard at my smoker practicing my brisket technique. I knew it could take me over the top in a barbecue contest.

The first things I had to learn were the basic facts about this cut. I'll make it easy for you: A whole brisket can be anywhere from 10 to 20 pounds. You'll probably have to order it from your local butcher because what's usually available in supermarket meat aisles is one of the two cuts that briskets are broken down into: flats and points. The first cut, or "the flat," comes from the area of the shoulder closest to the cow's belly and is evenly shaped and lean, while the narrow piece that's nearer to the fore-shank is rounder and fatter and is called "the point."

People ask me which cut of brisket is better, but the truth is they both have their advantages. The flat is easier to cook more consistently and evenly because of its shape; the point is preferred by some because it's often fattier and has more flavor. I'm going to give you two methods for cooking brisket, one for a whole brisket and the other for a flat, since these are the most common cuts available. It's likely you won't have to pick up your phone or log onto your computer to make a special order from the butcher because these are generally easy to find in the supermarket. If you find a "point," you can use the same method I'm giving you for the flat.

Smoked Brisket

If you want your brisket to turn out as delicious as possible, invest in quality meat. Anyone who has ever seen me cooking barbecue on TV knows that I favor wagyu beef, a type of cattle that has really fine marbling running through its meat, which means a lot of fat is interspersed with the muscle, and fat carries the flavor. Wagyu were first cultivated in Japan and have become known all over the world by all kinds of chefs and pitmasters for their rich flavor and tender, juicy flesh—which experts say comes from their grass-based diet. Here's the advice I give people who ask me whether it's worth it to spend the extra $30 on their briskets: Make two briskets side by side and judge the quality for yourself. I've never met anyone who did that and then went back to cooking cheaper meat. You will need a meat injector for this recipe. I use a 2-ounce "large capacity" stainless steel meat injector. (You can visit my website and buy one from me, if you like, at www.myronmixon.com.)

INGREDIENTS

15- to 20-pound whole untrimmed brisket, preferably wagyu beef

1 quart BBQ Keto Strong Beef Broth (*page 100*)

2 cups BBQ Beef Rub (*page 96*)

1. Following the directions under *Tips for Preparing Brisket for Smoking* (*page 109*), trim the brisket.

2. Once the brisket is trimmed, place it fat-side up in an aluminum baking pan. Load the beef injector with beef broth. Inject the brisket all over at 1-inch intervals; use about ¾ of the broth for injecting both sides of the brisket. Pour the remaining broth over the meat. Cover and refrigerate the meat in the aluminum baking pan for at least 6 to 8 hours or overnight.

3. About 30 minutes before you are ready to cook the brisket, heat a smoker to 350°F.

4. Remove the brisket from the fridge; discard the marinade and transfer the brisket to a cutting board. Use paper towels or a clean kitchen towel to pat the brisket dry thoroughly on both sides. Apply the rub all over the brisket on both sides, using your hands to rub it all over the meat. Transfer the brisket to a clean aluminum baking pan, place the pan in the smoker, and cook the brisket for 2½ hours.

5. After 2½ hours, remove the pan from the smoker and cover it with aluminum foil. Put it back on the smoker and cook it for another 1½ hours or until the temperature in the point-end of the meat reaches 205°F.

6. Remove the pan from the smoker. Discard the pan, wrap the brisket tightly with foil, and then wrap it in a thick blanket or large towel. Let the brisket rest this way for 3 or 4 hours.

7. Unwrap the brisket, discard the foil, and transfer the meat to a cutting board, taking care to save any juices that accumulated in the pan. (If you are going to make Burnt Ends, now is the time. (*See page 105*)

8. Strain the accumulated juices, and then transfer them to a medium saucepan. Warm the juices over medium heat and allow them to come to a gentle simmer but not a boil. While the juices gently simmer, slice the brisket against the grain into the size of slices that you like, taking care to cut consistently sized slices. Transfer the sliced brisket to a platter and pour the warm juices over the slices. Serve immediately.

Burnt Ends

After you have trimmed, marinated, smoked, and rested your brisket, if you want to make burnt ends you need to remove the bottom section of the brisket. Do this by locating the membrane that separates the bottom of the point (the narrow end of the brisket) from the top—it is visible, and you can feel it with the blade of your curved, narrow boning knife as you cut. Clean the fat from the membrane side of the bottom piece of brisket. Season the bottom piece with salt and pepper and then place it in an aluminum pan. Place the pan in the smoker and cook the bottom piece for 2 hours. After 2 hours, remove the burnt-end portion of the brisket from the smoker. Let it rest for 30 minutes. When finished resting, cut the meat into 1-inch cubes. Transfer the cubes to a small clean aluminum pan along with any drippings remaining in the original smoking pan. Cover the pan with aluminum foil and smoke the ends for an additional 30 minutes. Remove from the smoker and enjoy right away.

Backyard Brisket

SERVES 6 TO 8

Because brisket flats are often the most available form of brisket in supermarket meat cases, and because they cook in a manageable amount of time (6 to 8 hours) and are less work to prepare than whole briskets, many folks like to smoke them. The main thing you need to remember when you smoke one of these is that it's easy for the meat to dry out. The key to avoiding a dry brisket is to find an old blanket or thick towel and use it to wrap the foil-wrapped meat while it rests and its juices settle. I promise you that doing this will keep your brisket tender. Works for me every time.

INGREDIENTS

1 brisket flat, weighing 4½ to 5 pounds, with a layer of fat, ¼- to ½-inch thick

2 cups BBQ Beef Rub (*page 96*)

1. Use paper towels or a clean kitchen towel to pat the brisket thoroughly on both sides until dry. Apply the rub all over the brisket on both sides, using your hands to pat it (don't actually rub) all over the meat. Transfer the brisket to a clean aluminum baking pan, cover it with plastic wrap, and let it rest in the refrigerator for 4 to 6 hours before cooking.

2. An hour before you're ready to cook the brisket, remove the pan from the refrigerator.

3. Heat your smoker to 350°F.

4. Remove the plastic wrap from on top of the aluminum pan, place the pan in the smoker, and cook the brisket for 4 to 5 hours, until the internal temperature of the brisket reaches about 205°F. When the brisket reaches this temperature, remove the pan from the smoker and wrap the brisket first with aluminum foil, and then wrap it in a thick blanket or large towel. Let the brisket rest this way for 2 hours.

5. Unwrap the meat, discard the foil, and transfer the brisket to a cutting board, taking care to save any juices that accumulated in the pan. Strain the accumulated juices and then transfer them into a medium saucepan. Warm the juices over medium heat and allow them to come to a gentle simmer but do not boil. While the juices gently simmer, slice the brisket against the grain into the size of slices that you like, taking care to cut consistently sized slices. Transfer the slices to a platter and pour the warm juices over the slices. Serve immediately.

Tips for Preparing Brisket for Smoking

Before you cook a brisket, it's essential to trim the white-silvery web-like membrane of fat covering the meat. This is called the "silver." If you don't do this, the rub can't adhere to the meat, and the brisket will never become truly tender and flavorful. Your goal is to leave only ¼ inch of fat on the brisket. Removing the silver can be a painstaking process, but you need to take your time and do it right.

TIP 1: Brisket is much easier to trim when it's cold than when it's at room temperature, so trim it as soon as you take it out of the fridge.

TIP 2: Use a good, sharp, narrow curved boning knife for this task; a blunt blade is not going to do the job.

TIP 3: Put the brisket on a cutting board, fat cap up. Trim any bits of fat that are significantly thinner than the rest, because the thin pieces will cook too fast and burn. Trim the fat so it's uniformly about ¼-inch thick.

TIP 4: Turn the meat over to expose the silver. Poke the tip of the boning knife under the silver. Cut across the grain using a saw-like motion to remove the skin.

Beef Ribs

MAKES 8 RIBS, SERVES 4

I've been known to augment the English language with new, descriptive words in my time. I call these "Myronisms" and in my opinion they greatly improve communication, particularly when it comes to barbecue. One term I coined is "tenderlicious." I use it to describe beef ribs because there's simply no better way to describe these mini prime pieces of meat and bone that you can hold in your hands while you gnaw on all the good natural flavor they contain. Here's a tip for cooking beef ribs in particular: Do not over-season or over-sauce them. Sure, you want your ribs to be enhanced with flavoring agents, but these babies are already full of their own sweetness, and you don't want to mess too much with that.

INGREDIENTS

8 whole beef ribs, 2 racks, weighing 5 to 6 pounds total

2 tablespoons kosher salt

2 tablespoons ground black pepper

1 tablespoon monk fruit sweetener (*see page 19*)

1 teaspoon medium, mild, or hot chili powder

1 teaspoon ground turmeric

1 teaspoon ground coriander

1 teaspoon garlic powder

1 teaspoon onion powder

2 cups water

3½ cups Hickory BBQ Sauce (*page 99*)

1. The day before you want to cook the ribs, peel off the thick web-like membrane (or "silver") that covers the back side of each rib: Do this by working your fingers beneath the membrane until you have 2 to 3 inches cleared. Grab the membrane with a towel and pull gently but firmly away from the rib. (Or you can make your life easier and use one of my Rib Skinners that you can but at www.myronmixon.com.) Removing this silvery membrane exposes loose fat that will need trimming, so after you've peeled the membrane, use a paring or boning knife to cut off excess fat. Cut the rack into individual ribs, taking care to make each rib about the same size and with the same amount of meat on either side of the bone, if you can. Next use a clean kitchen towel or paper towels to pat the ribs dry. Set them aside on a cutting board or other clean surface.

2. In a medium bowl, combine the salt, pepper, monk fruit sweetener, chili powder, turmeric, coriander, garlic powder, and onion powder to form a rub. Coat both sides of each rib with the spice rub, rubbing the spices in with your fingers. Transfer the ribs to a large aluminum baking pan, cover with plastic wrap or aluminum foil, and refrigerate the pan overnight or at least for 6 to 8 hours.

recipe continues

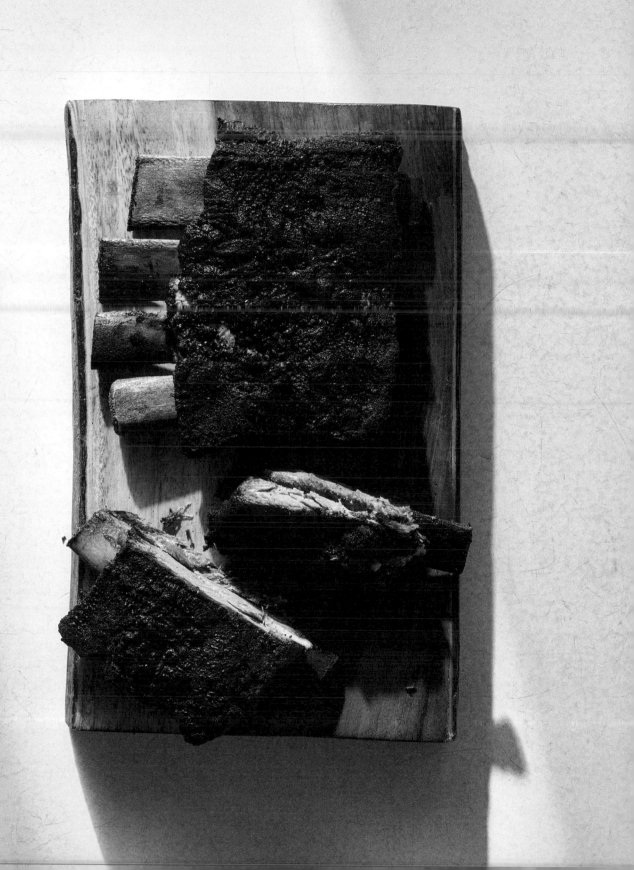

3. When you are ready to cook the ribs, heat a smoker to 275°F. When the smoker is ready, uncover the pan, place it in the smoker, and cook the ribs for 2 hours.

4. Remove the pan from the smoker and pour the water in the pan. Cover the pan with aluminum foil, return it to the smoker, and cook for 2 more hours.

5. Remove the ribs from the pan. Glaze the top side of the ribs with the Hickory BBQ Sauce. Don't overdo the sauce; use just enough to coat the ribs. Put the pan back in the smoker, uncovered, and cook for 15 minutes.

6. Remove the pan from the smoker and let the ribs sit, loosely covered, for 10 minutes. Now eat your ribs!

A Note About Ribs

When most of us think of "beef ribs" we picture the so-called Dinosaur Bones: the extra-long, heavy suckers that are loaded with chewy beef. In butchers' parlance, these are beef back ribs, meaning they are situated under the front section of a steer's backbone. These are a flavorful cut and often a good value for the money.

Not to be confused with what are labeled "beef ribs," short ribs, while still beef, are, as their name tells you, smaller than regular beef ribs. Short ribs is the term butchers use to describe cuts that come from the brisket chuck, "plate" (the belly just below the rib), or the actual ribs that feature a short portion of rib bone overlain by meat. The most common versions of short ribs look like palm-sized cubes, each with a little rib bone and a lot of meat. Some short ribs are also called "flanken" and are cut in a very different way from those called for here. Flanken are used a lot in Korean and Jewish cooking and are thin-cut horizontally from the front of the rib section, so they look like long, thin pieces of meat studded with many ribs—kind of like pieces of bacon, but with small bones in them. These are not the kind of ribs you want to smoke; save these for grilling as they don't need a long, slow cook.

Smoked Short Ribs

SERVES 4

A lot of cooks think you can only braise short ribs—they think that cooking them in liquid is the only way to make them tender. I disagree: If you know how to smoke short ribs, they can become tempting, tender, and kissed by the flavor of hickory smoke. Short ribs are prized by Keto diet folks like me because they're high in fat and full of rich beefy flavor.

INGREDIENTS

3 to 4 pounds bone-in beef short ribs, each 2 to 3 inches long (6 to 8 pieces)

¾ cup BBQ Beef Rub (*page 96*)

¾ cup Hickory BBQ Sauce (*page 99*)

1. Using paper towels or a clean kitchen towel, pat the short ribs dry all over. Generously coat the ribs with the rub, using your fingers to rub it in. Transfer the short ribs to a medium aluminum pan so they fit in a row, cover with plastic wrap, and refrigerate for at least 30 minutes and up to 6 or 7 hours.

2. When you're ready to smoke your short ribs, heat your smoker to 275°F. When the smoker is ready, uncover the pan, place it in the smoker, and cook the ribs for 2 hours.

3. Remove the pan from the smoker and pour 2 cups of water into the bottom of the pan. Cover the pan with the aluminum foil, return it to the smoker, and cook for 2 more hours.

4. Remove the ribs from the pan. Glaze the top side of the ribs with the Hickory BBQ Sauce only. Don't overdo it with the sauce; use just enough to coat the ribs. Put the pan back in the smoker, uncovered, and cook for 15 minutes.

5. Remove the pan from the smoker and let the ribs sit, loosely covered, for 10 minutes. Serve immediately.

Porterhouse Steaks with Lemony Tomato Sauce

SERVES 2

I've been married to my wife Faye for a long time, and I could not have achieved all that I have in the barbecue world without her by my side. We didn't have a whole lot when we first got together, but if we had, this is what I would've cooked for her on our first date. Nothing says "treat me right" like a porterhouse. The big hunk of steak combines two cuts. On one side of the bone is soft, rich tender-loin, and on the other side is firm and juicy sirloin. You want to splurge on your porterhouse. Buy top quality, which for me means wagyu but get the best that you can afford. And when you get a great porterhouse, take care to sear it long enough to develop a golden "crust" on the outside of the meat, which will lock in its big meaty flavors (a very, very hot grill or smoker helps). This is romance, people.

INGREDIENTS

FOR THE STEAKS:

1½-pound porterhouse steak, at least 1½ inches thick

1 cup BBQ Keto Strong Beef Broth (*page 100*)

Kosher salt

Ground black pepper

1 teaspoon onion powder

1 teaspoon garlic powder

FOR THE LEMONY TOMATO SAUCE:

½ cup pan juices from the steak or ½ cup BBQ Keto Strong Beef Broth (*page 100*) or another beef stock

8 tablespoons (1 stick) unsalted butter

¼ cup tomato paste

1 teaspoon monk fruit sweetener (*see page 19*)

2 teaspoons fresh lemon juice

FOR THE STEAKS:

1. Use paper towels or a clean kitchen towel to pat the steak dry all over. Place the steak in a baking dish, cover it with the cup of broth, cover the dish with plastic wrap, and marinate the steak at room temperature for 2 hours.

2. About 30 minutes before you're ready to cook the steak, heat your smoker or grill to 500°F.

3. Remove the steak from the marinade and discard the marinade. Season the steak liberally on both sides with salt and pepper. Sprinkle it with the onion powder and garlic powder.

4. When the smoker or grill is very hot, place the steak on the grill rack and sear it over direct heat for 3 to 4 minutes per side, depending on your preference for doneness (I sear them for 3 minutes to a side for medium rare).

5. Transfer the steak to a platter and cover it loosely with aluminum foil. Let it rest for 15 minutes.

FOR THE SAUCE:

1. Collect ¼ cup of the drippings from the platter where the steak is resting and pour them in a medium saucepan. If there are not enough drippings to measure ¼ cup, add beef broth until you have ¼ cup. Add the butter, tomato paste, monk fruit sweetener, and lemon juice. Over medium heat, whisk the sauce until the ingredients are well mixed and smooth. Let the sauce come to a boil and then immediately remove the pan from the heat and set aside to cool.

2. Uncover the steak and divide it between you and your lucky dining companion. First, use a sharp knife to remove the bone completely. (Don't toss it. Save it for later on, when you're alone in the kitchen and can gnaw away.) Cut the meat across the grain diagonally into thick, 1-inch slices. When you serve the steak, be sure to distribute meat from both sides of the steak. Pour the sauce over the slices. Enjoy immediately.

Smoked Bacon Cheeseburgers

MAKES 2 LARGE BURGERS

I love for my burgers to have that smoke-kissed flavor you can only get from cooking meat over wood inside an actual smoker. Nothing compares. If you're in a hurry, you can grill these bad boys instead of smoking them. Simply prepare a medium-hot fire in your grill, slide the burgers on a rack directly over the hot coals, cover the grill, and cook the burgers for 5 to 7 minutes per side for medium rare (about 145°F). But if you have the time, try my old-school way for smoking; I promise these are worth firing up your wood box. They are that good.

INGREDIENTS

1 pound ground beef, the freshest and best quality you can find

3 tablespoons BBQ Beef Rub (*page 96*)

2 tablespoons Pitmaster's Buttermilk Ranch Dressing Mix (*page 163*)

2 tablespoons unsalted butter

2 slices sharp cheddar cheese

4 large iceberg lettuce leaves, plus more for topping the burgers

4 slices bacon

1 medium-size tomato, sliced

1. In a medium bowl, combine the ground beef with the rub and the ranch mix, just until the spices are integrated with the beef. Take care not to overhandle the meat. Form the meat into 2 equal-size patties (you can make more burgers if you like smaller ones, but I don't). Transfer the burgers to a shallow aluminum pan, cover with plastic wrap, and refrigerate until ready to cook.

2. Heat your smoker to 300°F.

3. Remove the burgers from the refrigerator, uncover, discard the plastic wrap, and place the pan in the smoker. Cook for 15 minutes for medium-rare (about 145°F) or up to 30 minutes for medium-well (about 155°F).

4. Remove the burgers from the smoker and allow them to rest in their pan, uncovered, while you melt the butter in a medium skillet over medium heat. When the butter is hot but not smoking, use a spatula to slide the burgers carefully into the skillet. Sear the burgers for about 3 minutes on each side or just until a golden-brown crust has formed—be careful not to overcook them. Slide the burgers onto a plate and immediately top them with slices of cheddar cheese. Cover the plate loosely with aluminum foil to let the cheeseburgers rest and the cheese melt.

recipe continues

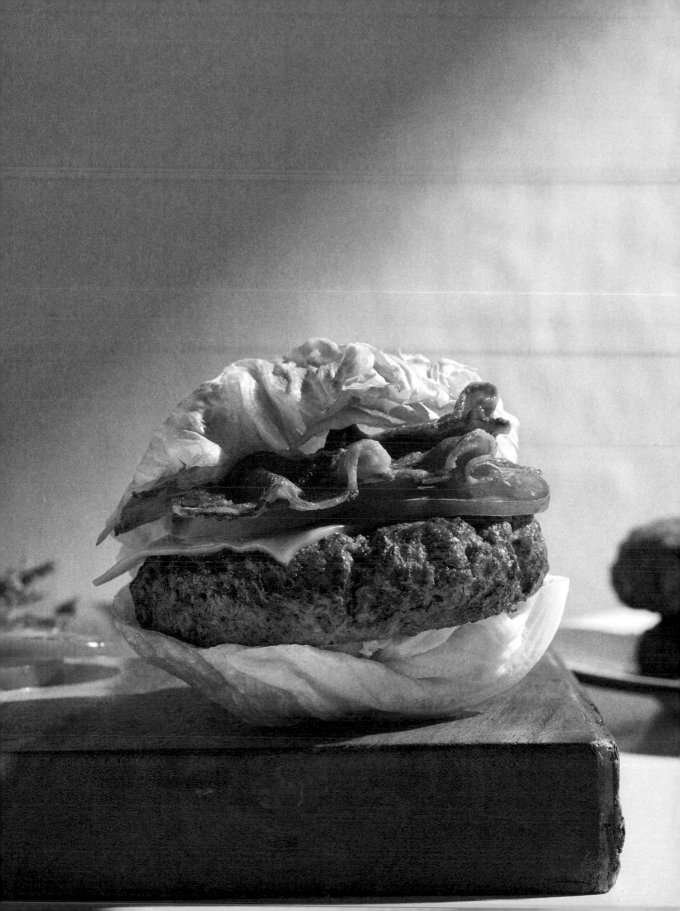

5. While the burgers are resting, cook the bacon to your desired crispness.

6. Lay overlapping lettuce leaves on a platter or similar dish. Place the burgers on them. Top each with two slices of bacon and tomato slices. Cover the burgers with additional lettuce leaves to create a "bun." Belleve me when I tell you, after you taste these you will not miss that cottony old bun one bit.

Beef Tenderloin

SERVES 6

If a brisket had an opposite, it might well be a beef tenderloin. This is a very delicate and tender cut and if cooked right will have a lovely soft texture. A tenderloin is so tender because the meat comes from the area along the rear portion of a cow's spine, right behind the kidney and running from the hip to the lower rib; an area, in other words, that doesn't get a lot of working out or exercise. This meat does not need an injection of moisture to make it delicious; as its name tells you, it's tender already. Your job is not to screw it up. Do not overcook this meat. It is meant to be cooked no more than medium-rare for optimal results. If that doesn't sound good to you, skip it and cook something that suffers less from being well done—more tenderloin for me that way. By all means shell out for a tenderloin if you're cooking for people who you want to impress.

INGREDIENTS

3 pounds beef tenderloin roast

4 cups BBQ Keto Strong Beef Broth (*page 100*)

½ cup distilled white vinegar

⅓ cup monk fruit sweetener (*see page 19*)

12-ounce can club soda

1. Use a clean kitchen towel or paper towels to thoroughly pat the tenderloin dry. Combine the broth, vinegar, monk fruit sweetener, and club soda in a gallon-size sealable plastic bag. Submerge the tenderloin in this marinade, seal the bag so it is airtight, and refrigerate overnight or for at least 6 to 8 hours.

2. When you are ready to cook the tenderloin, heat a smoker to 275°F.

3. Transfer the tenderloin to a clean aluminum roasting plan and discard the marinade. Put the pan in the smoker and cook for about 1½ hours, or until the internal temperature at the center of the tenderloin reaches 155°F on a digital meat thermometer. Transfer the tenderloin to a cutting board and let it rest for 15 minutes.

4. When ready to serve, cut the tenderloin crosswise into ½-inch thick slices and serve immediately.

Smoked Beef Stew

SERVES 6 TO 8

Sometimes people are surprised when they discover the variety of dishes I like to put in my smoker. Before I lost a ton of weight on Keto and became as svelte as I am today, I used to bake a chocolate cake in my smoker. Those days are over, but I tell you what: A delicious smoked beef stew on a cold winter night will give you the warm and fuzzies.

INGREDIENTS

2½ pounds beef chuck roast, cut into 1½-inch cubes

2 tablespoons BBQ Beef Rub (*page 96*)

Kosher salt and freshly ground black pepper

2 tablespoons butter

3½ cups BBQ Keto Strong Beef Broth (*page 100*)

1 small white onion, chopped

4 cloves garlic, minced

1 tablespoon tomato paste

1 tablespoon Hickory BBQ Sauce (*page 99*)

2 teaspoons dried thyme

2 stalks celery, sliced

1 medium carrot, peeled and cut into rounds

OPTIONAL: ½ cup full-fat sour cream or full-fat cream (to thicken stew), minced flatleaf parsley, ½ cup grated sharp cheddar cheese

1. In a medium bowl combine the beef cubes with the rub, salt, and pepper. Use your hands to coat the cubes.

2. Over medium heat, melt the butter in a heavy stockpot, taking care not to let it burn. Add about ¼ of the beef cubes to the pot and let them brown on all sides, turning them as they cook. Remove the batch of cubes before adding the next. When all the beef is browned, return it to the stockpot and pour in the broth. Use a wooden or another spoon to stir and scrape up any flavorful browned bits sticking to the bottom of the pot. Turn the heat to low and stir in the onion, garlic, tomato paste, Hickory BBQ Sauce, and thyme. Cover the pot with a lid, remove it from the heat, and set aside.

3. Heat the smoker to 300°F.

4. Transfer the stew from the Dutch oven, or whatever container you used, to a medium aluminum baking pan. Cover it tightly with aluminum foil and place it in the smoker. Let the stew cook for 2 hours. Remove the stew from the smoker, uncover, and add the celery and carrots. Cover again, return to the smoker, and continue to cook for about 2 hours longer over low heat.

5. When ready to serve, transfer the stew to bowls. If the stew isn't very thick, you can add full-fat sour cream. If you'd like, top with minced fresh parsley or with some grated cheddar cheese.

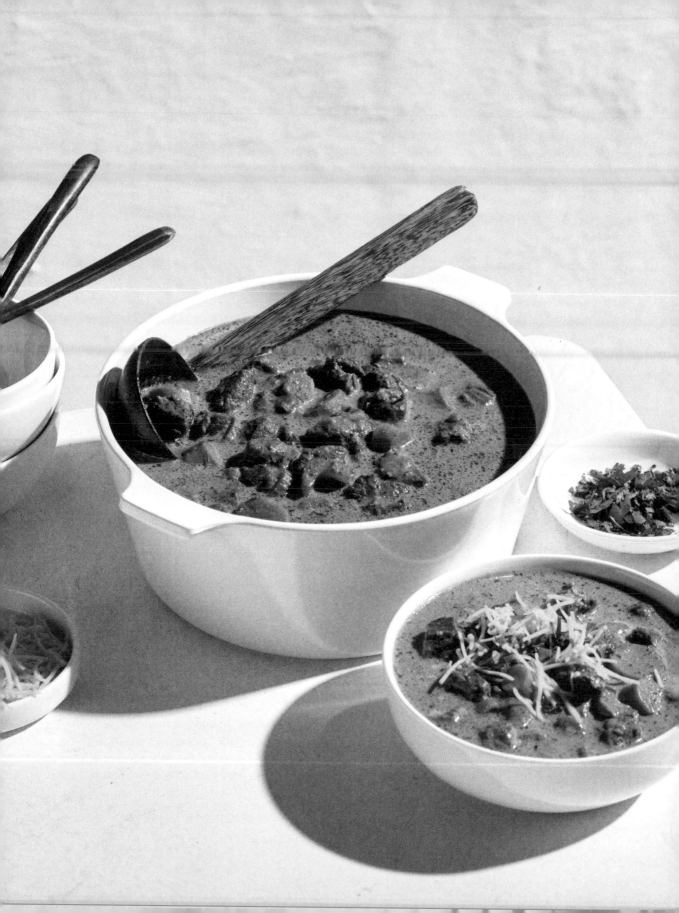

Prime Rib Fit for a King

SERVES 6 TO 8

To me nothing says decadence like prime rib. It's a primal cut of beef, meaning that it's one that is separated from the steer during its initial butchering and not after that. The rib just naturally has a lot of intramuscular fat, a.k.a. marbling, which makes it ideal for the Keto lifestyle. You might say prime rib and me go well together. Prime rib is the king of all beef cuts, and I'm the king of barbecue. It's also expensive and you'll be asked to pay good money for it, so you want to be sure you take care to make it as delicious as possible. But one reason it is worth it, besides the fact that it tastes great, is that with this roast there's something for everyone on it: The ends are going to be more well done and the center is going to be bright pink. By the way, you will need a meat injector for this recipe.

INGREDIENTS

3-rib standing rib roast, weighing 7 pounds and well marbled

1 recipe BBQ Keto Strong Beef Broth (page 100)

Kosher salt and ground black pepper

1 tablespoon onion powder

2 tablespoons garlic powder

1. Use a clean kitchen towel or paper towels to pat the roast dry all over. Place the roast in an aluminum roasting pan. Load your beef injector with cool broth; inject the roast all over at 1-inch-square intervals. Cover the pan with plastic wrap or aluminum foil and refrigerate the roast overnight or for at least 6 to 8 hours.

2. When you are ready to cook the roast, heat a smoker to 250°F.

3. Transfer the roast from the pan to a cutting board. Use a clean kitchen towel or paper towels to pat the roast dry all over. Season the roast with salt, pepper, onion powder, and garlic powder, gently rubbing the spices into the meat. Put the roast back in the pan and put the pan in the smoker. Cook for 5 hours or until the internal temperature reaches 155°F at the center of the roast.

4. Take the roast out of the smoker. Transfer it to a clean roasting pan and cover with aluminum foil. Wrap the pan in a thick blanket or towel and let it rest at room temperature for 1 hour.

5. Unwrap the pan and transfer the roast to a cutting board. Pour the drippings in the pan into a medium saucepan set over medium heat. Bring the drippings to a simmer, reduce the heat, and cook gently for 5 minutes without coming to a boil. Pour the heated drippings over the roast. Carve it and serve it immediately.

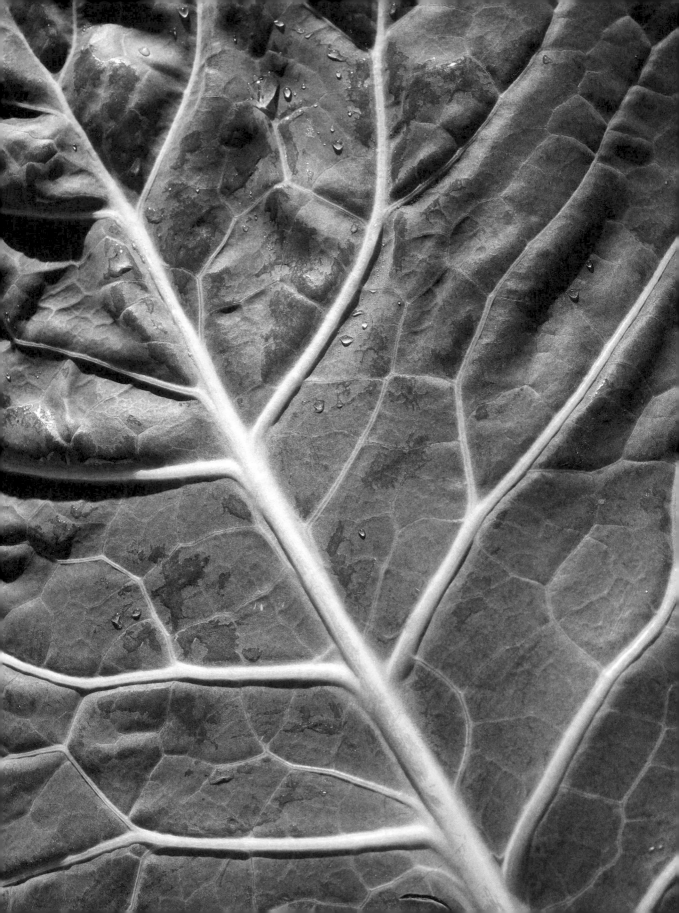

CHAPTER 5

Vegetables & Greens
(yeah, you eat them, too)

IN THIS CHAPTER, I emphasize how to make the traditional barbecue plate's "two sides," the healthful part of the meal. I used to be a person who wanted to run away at the thought of "healthy sides" and used eating barbecue as a way to deliver carbs. To me, sides were supposed to up the ante on the plate by giving you something fried or starchy to sop up the meat and any juices. That's really what I used to think. I don't think that anymore, though. Now that I know what my body needs to be healthy, thanks to the Keto diet, I look at side dishes very differently. And I have figured out how to make my barbecue sides even better because of this reconsideration.

When it comes to barbecue, side dishes have always been important. I don't have time for those folks who claim nobody cares about side dishes. I do, and our families and friends always have. I remember my granny cooking all the classic Southern sides for our family's dinners: potato salad, coleslaw, baked beans, you name it. So, my challenge became figuring out how to replicate those classics in a way that was in keeping with my Keto plan. For example, I don't have potato salad—but I do still have a delicious version of "tater tots" that I rely on whenever I feel like having something indulgent with my pulled pork.

At the most basic level, what we want our barbecue sides to do is complement the smoky sweetness of the meat. Some barbecue contests actually have competitions for side dishes, which shows you how seriously pitmasters take all of our food, not just the main event. And one thing I've learned from winning a few of those competitions is that people like their side dishes to be plentiful and recognizable. For example, nobody is looking for the world's most modern and innovative coleslaw. You want coleslaw to be creamy, crunchy, and tangy—the kind that's going to balance the meat's rich flavors.

It's true that you have to give up potato-based sides on Keto. You know what I say to that? Who cares! You don't need French fries to have a great barbecue, never have and never will. I'm here to offer you a host of options for healthy side dishes to go with all your favorite grilled and smoked meats. What is more, I'm here to do it in a way that is going to keep your Keto going and keep you looking and feeling your best, without packing on the pounds.

RECLES

Pitmaster's Smoky Collards and Kale

SERVES 4 TO 6

My granny cooked collards in a classic way that'll be recognizable to all my Southerners out there: low and slow in a big pot, with pork to add some salt and fat to the greens. In my version, I cook the bacon until it's almost crisp but not quite, then let the drippings, onions, and garlic add a smoky essence to them. The paprika and crushed red pepper bring a little heat, and the vinegar brings the tang. I'm lucky that this traditional formula for Southern-style greens is a perfect fit for the Keto diet. Make sure to take note of the fact that greens are finished cooking when they're shiny: My granny's greens were known for their shine, and I pride mine on the same criteria.

INGREDIENTS

1½ pounds collard greens, about 2 bunches

1 pound leafy green kale

2 tablespoons olive oil

8 ounces bacon, cut into 1½-inch pieces

1 medium yellow onion, diced

4 cloves garlic, diced

2 teaspoons smoked paprika

1 teaspoon crushed red pepper flakes

½ cup red wine

¼ cup apple cider vinegar

2 cups BBQ Keto Strong Beef Broth (*page 100*) or store-bought beef stock

Kosher salt and pepper

1. Wash all the greens well in cold water. Trim your collards and your kale greens with a sharp knife. Remove the center rib from each leaf. Discard the ribs and then cut the greens into thin strips and set them aside.

2. In a large pot set over medium-low heat, heat the olive oil and then add the bacon strips, cooking the bacon just until soft and translucent; do not brown. Add the onion and continue to sauté the bacon with the onion until the bacon begins to crisp and brown around the edges and the onion pieces are translucent and soft. Add the garlic and cook for 1 to 2 minutes, just until fragrant. Do not let the garlic burn. Add the paprika and pepper flakes. Cook for 30 seconds, stirring, taking care not to let the spices burn. Pour in the red wine and deglaze the bottom of the pan by scraping up any bits of bacon, onions, or garlic that have stuck to the bottom of the pan. Add the vinegar and stock and bring to a simmer. Add the greens to the pot. Stir and cover the pot to allow the greens to wilt for 10 minutes. Uncover, stir again to combine, and reduce the heat to low.

3. Let the greens slowly simmer for 1 hour, stirring occasionally. If all the liquid seems to be evaporating, add extra stock or water as needed, ½ cup at a time. The greens are finished cooking when the leaves are tender, shiny, and almost all the liquid evaporates. Season with salt and pepper, if you'd like, and serve.

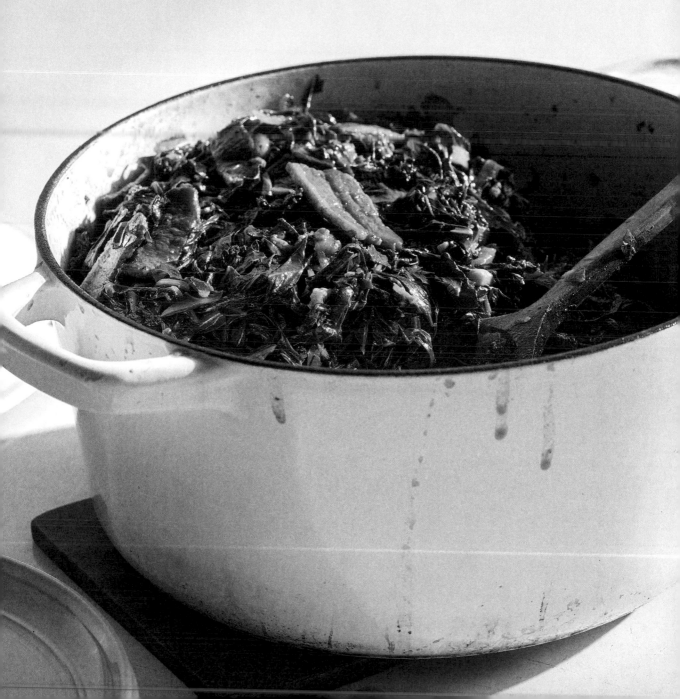

Mama's Classic Slaw

SERVES 4 TO 6

If I had to choose just one essential side dish for barbecue, it would be this one. The cool creaminess of this slaw paired with the hot meat fresh out of the smoker—well, that's heaven on a plate right there. I know the world is filled with all kinds of new ways of making slaw from things like Brussels sprouts (look, even I do it; see page 132), but for the times when nothing but the classic version will do, this is where you should turn. I also love this with a fish fry (even though I don't batter my fish in flour any more these days).

INGREDIENTS

¼ cup mayonnaise (be sure to choose a brand with no added sugar)

¼ cup full fat sour cream

¼ cup heavy cream

4 tablespoons fresh lemon juice or apple cider vinegar, or a combination

1 teaspoon Dijon mustard

1 teaspoon celery salt

1 tablespoon BBQ Beef Rub (*page 96*)

1 pound shredded red and green cabbage

1. In a large mixing bowl, whisk together all of the ingredients, except the cabbage.

2. Add the shredded cabbage and toss to combine and coat the greens thoroughly. Cover and chill for at least 1 hour before serving. You can make this up to 1 day ahead of time. Refrigerate until serving.

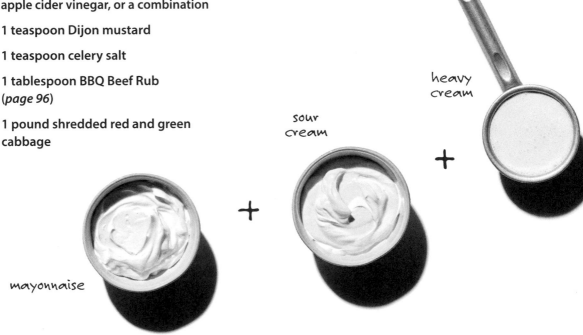

mayonnaise + sour cream + heavy cream

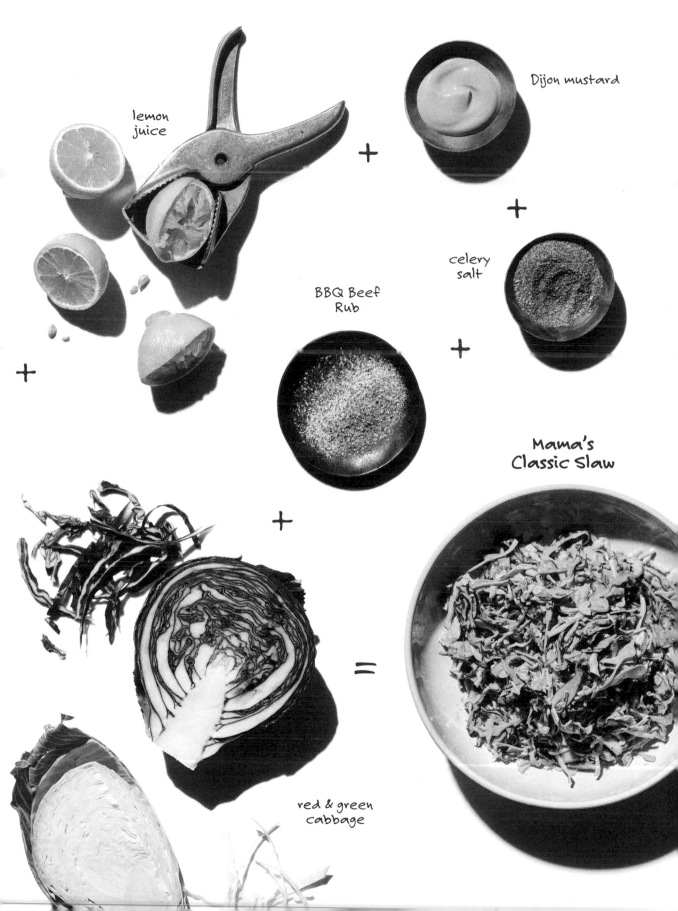

lemon juice

Dijon mustard

+

+

celery salt

BBQ Beef Rub

+

+

+

red & green cabbage

=

Mama's Classic Slaw

Brussels Sprouts Slaw with Blue Cheese, Bacon, and Pecans

SERVES 4 TO 6

Nowadays you can buy Brussels sprouts already shredded, but if you can't find those in your local supermarket just shred up your sprouts in a food processor fitted with a slicing blade (not the knife blade or the shredder). All you have to do is push the sprouts through to create thin ribbons. This is a great counterbalance to fork-tender pulled pork because it's triple crunchy: you get the sprouts, the pecans, and the bacon to chomp on.

INGREDIENTS

⅓ cup olive oil

2 tablespoons fresh lemon juice

1 tablespoon Dijon mustard

1 teaspoon garlic powder

1 teaspoon kosher salt

½ teaspoon black pepper

1 pound Brussels sprouts, thinly shaved or finely chopped

6 slices cooked, crispy bacon, crumbled

½ cup chopped pecans

¼ cup crumbled blue cheese

1. In a large bowl, whisk together the olive oil, lemon juice, mustard, garlic powder, salt, and black pepper. Add the shredded sprouts and toss to coat. Add the bacon crumbles, pecans, and blue cheese. Toss well. Cover and chill for at least 1 hour before serving. You can make this up to 1 day ahead of time. Refrigerate until serving.

Smoked Cabbage

SERVES 6

This smoky head of cabbage is a pitmaster's version of sauerkraut and is easy to make because you can slide it into the smoker right alongside whatever you're already smoking. I wouldn't advise anyone to fire up their smoker just to cook this cabbage, but I would suggest that any time you're already smoking something, you toss on a head of this seasoned cabbage. When it's done, it's buttery, smoky, and tangy—just right with brisket, ribs, chicken wings, you name it.

INGREDIENTS

**8 tablespoons butter
(1 stick), softened**

**2 tablespoons BBQ Beef Rub
(page 96)**

1 head green cabbage

1. In a small bowl, use a fork to mix the softened butter with the rub.

2. Core the green cabbage by carving out a good-size cavity in the center, taking care not to cut all the way through the leaves. Leave about a 1-inch shell. Stuff the seasoned butter into the cabbage cavity. Wrap the cabbage completely in heavy-duty aluminum foil and put the cabbage, cored-end up, on the top rack of the smoker.

3. Close the lid and smoke the cabbage until soft, at least 3 hours and up to 4, depending on the temperature of the smoker and how many other things you might be smoking in it at the same time. Unwrap the cabbage and discard any blackened leaves. Cut the cabbage into wedges and serve.

Pitmaster Iceberg Wedge Salad with Bacon

SERVES 4

Everybody knows that a wedge salad's main function is to deliver blue cheese and bacon to your belly. I like my wedge served up steakhouse-style, with cherry tomatoes, hardboiled eggs, and a few scallions scattered here and there. This is my "desert island" first course, a number-one personal favorite and 100% Keto.

INGREDIENTS

1 head iceberg lettuce

3 hardboiled eggs, diced

4 slices crispy, cooked bacon, crumbled

4 scallions, sliced, white and light green parts only

½ cup halved cherry tomatoes

1 cup Blue Cheese Dressing (*page 164*)

1. Wash the head of lettuce in cold water and remove and discard any damaged or brown outer leaves. Use a sharp knife to cut the head into 4 equally sized wedges.

2. Divide the wedges among 4 salad plates, placing them with the outer leaves down. Divide the eggs, bacon, scallions, and tomatoes evenly among the wedges, sprinkling them over the top of the lettuce. Dress each salad by spooning ¼ cup of the blue cheese dressing over the top of each.

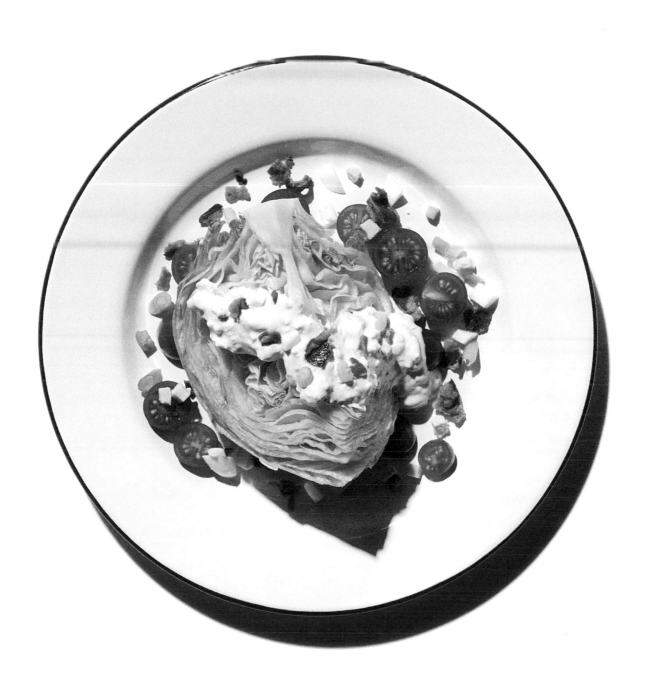

Smoked Broccoli with Parm and Lemon

SERVES 6 TO 8

A seldom-reported fact about pitmasters is that we do eat green vegetables. I once heard somebody say that broccoli is America's favorite. I like it, but I especially like it after it's been kissed by smoke, seasoned with barbecue rub, and topped with a good-size grate of parm (Parmesan cheese). I'll bet you haven't tried it this way yet, but you'll thank me after you do.

INGREDIENTS

1¼ pounds broccoli crowns, cut into florets (about 8 cups)

3 tablespoons fresh lemon juice

3 tablespoons olive oil

3 cloves garlic, minced

2 tablespoons BBQ Beef Rub (*page 96*)

⅓ cup grated Parmesan cheese

1. Place the broccoli in a large plastic bag. Whisk together the lemon juice, oil, garlic, and rub and drizzle over the broccoli. Toss to coat and set aside for 30 minutes.

2. When ready to cook in your smoker, transfer the broccoli to a medium-size aluminum pan. Cover the pan loosely with foil and smoke it for 30 minutes. After 30 minutes, remove the cover and continue to smoke for 15 minutes longer. Remove the pan from the smoker, top the broccoli with the Parmesan, and serve immediately.

3. To make this in the oven instead of the smoker, pre-heat the oven to 450°F. When ready to cook, transfer the broccoli to a rimmed baking sheet and arrange it in a single layer. Roast until the broccoli begins to brown, about 8 minutes. Remove from the oven, toss with the Parmesan, and serve immediately.

Veggie Kebabs

SERVES 8

Here's the deal. To make really good vegetable kebabs, you need to grill each vegetable on its own skewer. Don't mix them up and put a few different vegetables on the skewers. It might look cool that way because it's more colorful, but the only right way to ensure that the vegetables are cooked consistently and evenly is to use a different skewer (or skewers) for each vegetable. And then if you still want things to look colorful, arrange the skewers that way when you serve them. You will need 18 (12-inch) metal or wooden skewers (if using wooden skewers, soak them in warm water for 30 minutes before using). You can grill any vegetables you like, but these are my favorites.

INGREDIENTS

FOR THE VINAIGRETTE:

½ cup apple cider vinegar

1 tablespoon balsamic vinegar

1 large garlic clove, minced

1 cup olive oil

2 teaspoons BBQ Beef Rub (*page 96*)

1 teaspoon kosher salt

¼ teaspoon monk fruit sweetener (*see page 19*)

FOR THE VEGETABLES:

1 pound zucchini, cut into ¾-inch-thick slices

¾ pound cherry tomatoes

1 pound baby eggplant, about 4 inches long and cut crosswise into ¾-inch-thick slices

10 ounces white button mushrooms, trimmed

2 red bell peppers, cut into 1½-inch pieces

1 large red onion, cut into 1½-inch pieces

Olive oil

BBQ Beef Rub (*page 96*)

recipe continues

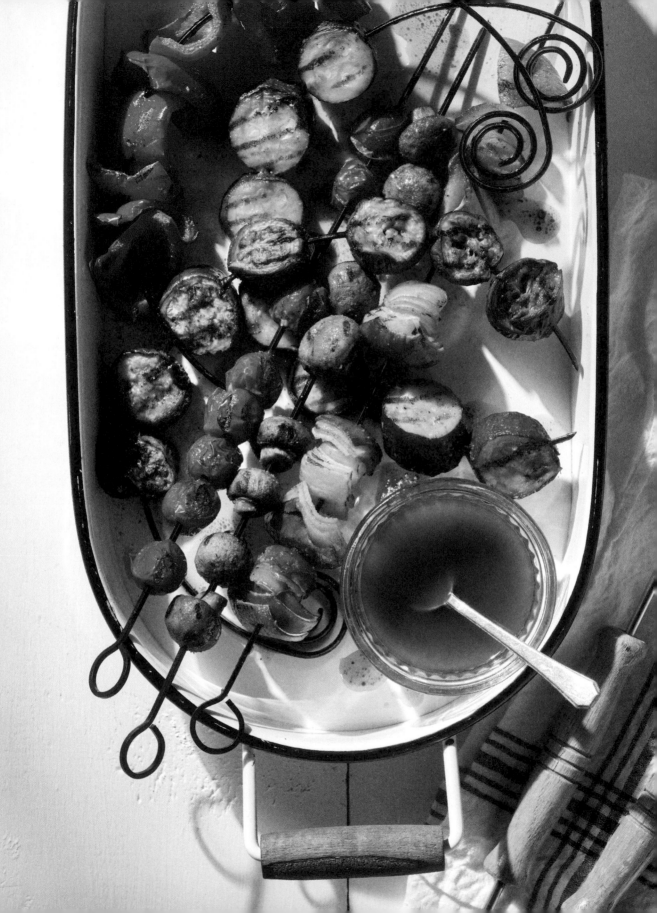

1. First make the vinaigrette: whisk together all the vinaigrette ingredients until combined.

2. Prepare the grill for cooking over medium-hot charcoal (moderate heat for gas grills).

3. To prepare the vegetables for grilling, put the zucchini in a large bowl with 2 teaspoons of oil and the rub. Toss to mix. Thread the coated vegetables on the skewers. Repeat with the remaining vegetables, working with one type at a time and keeping each vegetable on skewers with vegetables of the same type. All vegetables should be coated lightly in olive oil and with the rub when you are finished.

   TIPS:
   - You can thread the zucchini and eggplant horizontally through the slices so the cut sides will lie flat on the grill.
   - When you thread the tomatoes, mushrooms, bell peppers, and onions, leave about ¾ inch between each one.
   - You should end up using 3 skewers per type of vegetable, and not mixing vegetables on any skewer.

4. When all the vegetables are threaded onto skewers, grill the kebabs in two batches on a lightly oiled grill rack (covered only if using a gas grill), turning over once until the vegetables are tender and all but the tomatoes are lightly browned. The tomatoes should blister and shrivel. The total time should be 6 to 10 minutes, but it will vary among vegetables. Pull off each vegetable when it's done. Don't wait for all of them to be done, as you'll end up ruining those that cook quicker.

5. Transfer the skewers to a platter. Drizzle them with the vinaigrette and serve immediately.

Buffalo BBQ Brussels Sprouts

SERVES 4

This recipe may just be proof that there is no food that can't be made Buffalo-style. The familiar hot sauce and blue cheese combo is excellent when you apply it to some butter-roasted tiny heads of cabbage. This is something I would not have tried if not for Keto, but now it's an easy weeknight side dish for us, a standby that goes with anything I pull off the smoker.

INGREDIENTS

5 tablespoons olive oil

1 pound Brussels sprouts, trimmed and halved

2 teaspoons BBQ Beef Rub (*page 96*)

2 garlic cloves, minced

¼ cup hot sauce

1 tablespoon fresh lemon juice

¼ cup (½ stick) unsalted butter, chilled and cubed

Kosher salt and ground pepper

¼ cup blue cheese crumbles

1. Preheat the oven to 400°F.

2. In a large ovenproof skillet, heat 4 tablespoons of the olive oil over medium-high heat. Add the Brussels sprouts and cook, stirring as needed, until golden, about 3 to 4 minutes. Season with the rub.

3. Place the skillet in the oven and cook until the Brussels sprouts are tender, 5 to 6 minutes longer. Transfer the sprouts to a bowl and return the skillet to medium heat.

4. Add the remaining 1 tablespoon of olive oil and the garlic to the pan. Cook until the garlic is lightly golden, 1 to 2 minutes. Add the hot sauce and lemon juice and remove the pan from the heat.

5. Whisk in the butter until thoroughly combined, about 1 minute, and then stir in the Brussels sprouts. Season with salt and pepper. Transfer the Brussels sprouts to a platter. Top with blue cheese crumbles and serve immediately.

Smoked Garlic Butter Mushrooms

SERVES 4 TO 6

I tell folks who are just getting interested in smoking meats that they can expand their horizons and try smoking just about anything else they like to eat—for example, mushrooms. These make a decadent side dish for grilled steaks and for smoked brisket; the meaty, earthy flavors of these mushrooms stand up to the richness of the beef. You can also stick a few toothpicks in these suckers and pass them around with cocktails as an hors d'oeuvres—a pitmaster's version of the fifties classic, stuffed mushrooms, but without the mushy stuffing and with plenty of smoky garlic butter in its place.

INGREDIENTS

4 cups baby bella mushrooms

2 tablespoons butter, melted

1 teaspoon garlic powder

1 teaspoon salt

1 teaspoon pepper

OPTIONAL: flat-leaf parsley, chopped

1. Using a mushroom brush or pastry brush or just your fingers and a paper towel, gently brush any dirt off the mushrooms and clean them as well as you can.

2. In a medium bowl, combine the melted butter and the seasonings. Gently toss in the mushrooms, making sure to coat them with the butter mixture while not letting them tear. Transfer the mushrooms to a medium aluminum pan and spread them out so they're not sitting on top of one another.

3. When ready to cook, preheat the smoker to 250°F.

4. Place the pan containing the mushrooms in the smoker. Smoke the mushrooms in the pan for 30 minutes.

5. Serve the mushrooms warm with a little chopped parsley on top, if you like.

Garlicky Mashed Cauliflower

SERVES 4

This is your straight-up more nutritious but just-as-comforting Keto version of mashed potatoes. I know, I was dubious at first, too. But I like the nutty flavor, and the fact that no matter how much you mash your cauliflower it won't ever turn gummy like the potato version sometimes does. You can find "riced" cauliflower in a lot of supermarkets nowadays and you're welcome to sub it in this recipe. 2 pounds of riced cauliflower equals 1 large head of fresh cauliflower.

INGREDIENTS

8 cups bite-size cauliflower florets (about 2 medium-size heads of cauliflower)

4 large cloves garlic, crushed

⅓ cup full fat sour cream

4 teaspoons olive oil

2 teaspoons unsalted butter

2 teaspoons salt

Freshly ground black pepper

OPTIONAL: fresh chives or parsley (or your favorite herbs), chopped

1. Place the cauliflower florets and garlic in a steamer basket set over boiling water, cover and steam until very tender, 12 to 15 minutes. (Alternatively, place florets and garlic in a microwave-safe bowl with ¼ cup water, cover, and microwave on high for 3 to 5 minutes until tender.)

2. Transfer the cooked cauliflower and garlic to a food processor. Add the sour cream, 2 teaspoons of oil, butter, salt, and pepper. Pulse several times, and then process until smooth and creamy. Transfer to a serving bowl. Drizzle the remaining 2 teaspoons of oil over the cauliflower. If you'd like, garnish with chives or parsley or your favorite herbs. Serve piping hot.

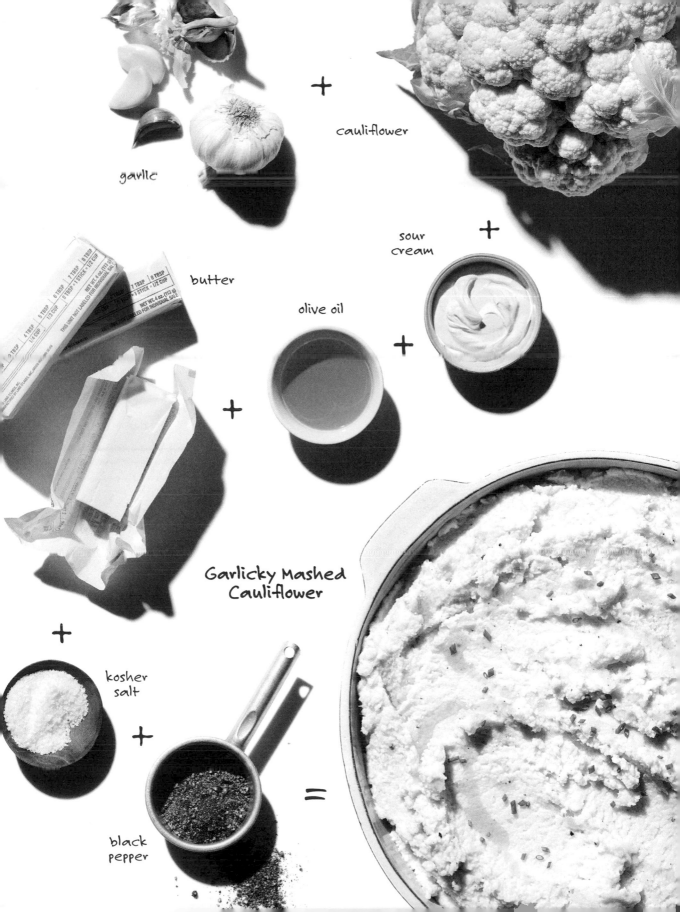

garlic

+

cauliflower

+

butter

olive oil

sour
cream

+

+

**Garlicky Mashed
Cauliflower**

+

kosher
salt

+

black
pepper

=

Keto "Tater Tots"

SERVES 4

While I don't much care for fake noodles made out of zucchini, I gotta tell you that I do find zucchini is a great substitute for one of my favorite guilty pleasures: tater tots. Yep, from the old lunchroom trays of my youth. I know you love 'em, too. If you make them with grated zucchini, plenty of parm and some barbecue rub, they'll be the best tots you ever put in your mouth. Give it a shot.

INGREDIENTS

3 medium zucchinis, grated

Yolks of 2 large eggs, lightly beaten (reserve whites for something else)

½ cup shredded cheddar cheese

1 cup grated Parmesan cheese

1 teaspoon BBQ Beef Rub (*page 96*)

1 teaspoon dried oregano

Kosher salt and freshly ground black pepper

1. Grease a rimmed baking sheet with cooking spray. Working over the kitchen sink, wrap the grated zucchini into a bowl. Transfer to cheese cloth or several paper towels or a clean kitchen towel and squeeze all excess water out of it. Keep wringing to get the zucchini shreds as dry as possible. This step is important. You have to get as much of the liquid out as you can or your tots will never be crispy.

2. In a large bowl, mix together the grated zucchini with the beaten egg yolks, cheeses, rub, and oregano.

3. Using a tablespoon as a measure, spoon about 1 tablespoon of the mixture into your hand and roll it between your palms into a tater-tot shape. These tater tots are rectangular little pillows of veggies, each 1½ to 2 inches long, or larger if you prefer. Repeat the process with the rest of the mixture until your pan is lined with tots. Refrigerate the tots for 20 minutes.

4. Preheat the oven to 400°F.

5. Bake the tots for 15 to 20 minutes, or until golden. Season with salt and pepper. Serve immediately.

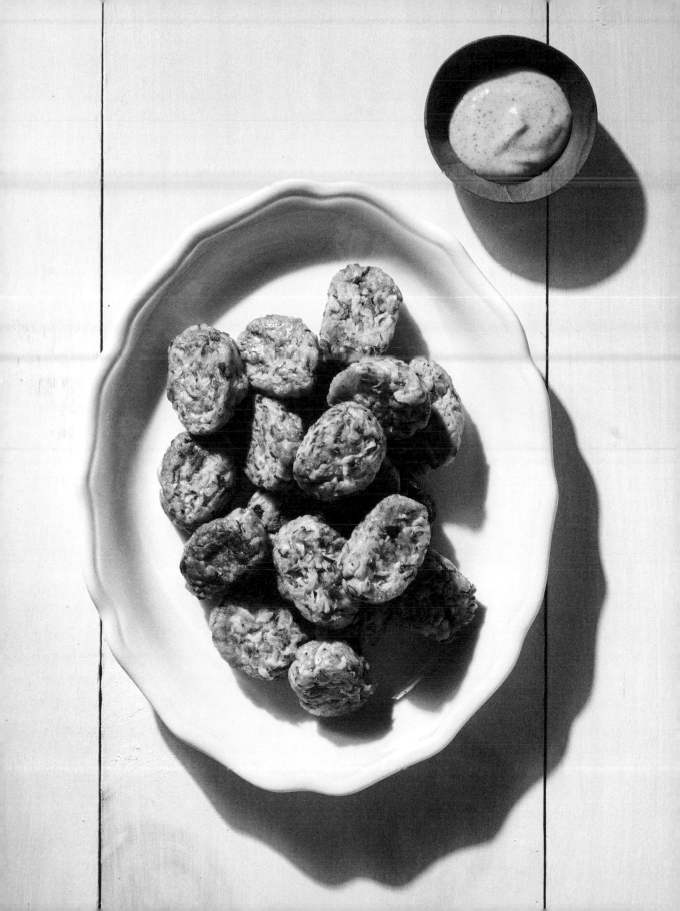

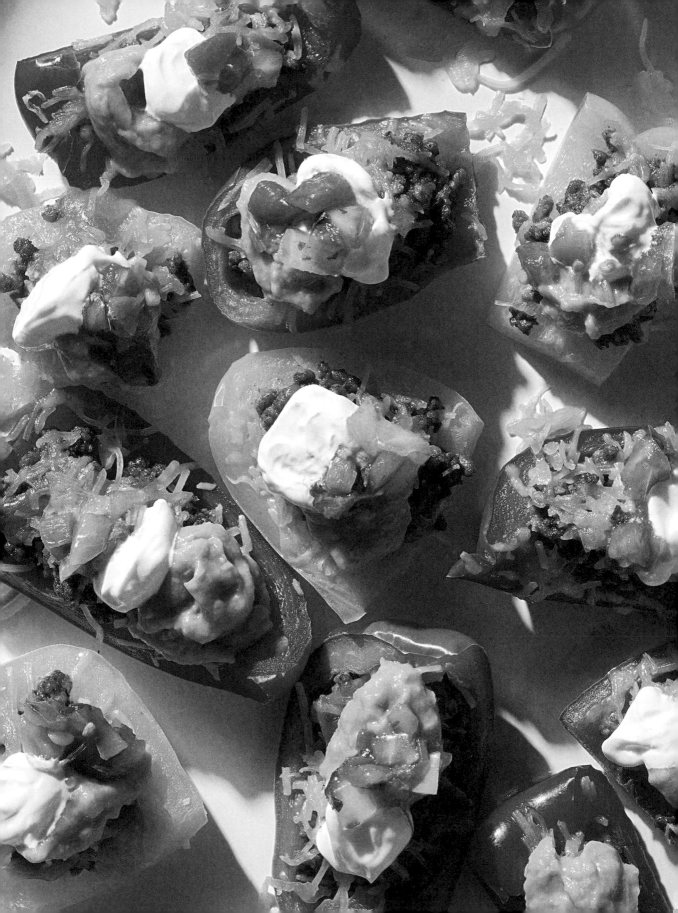

CHAPTER 6

Apps & Snacks

I'M GOING TO BE HONEST WITH YOU. I have a favorite snack, and it is not in this chapter. It's not even in this book. There isn't even a recipe for it. Why? Because it's a bowl of blackberries. Sometimes I pour a little cream on top of them, but mostly I don't. If I'm not at a barbecue cooking competition or on the road doing a cooking demo or making a tv show, you can find me walking around my house or my outdoor barbecue pavilion carrying a bowl of blackberries in my hand. I love this tart'n'tangy fruit, and it's perfect for Keto. Just cutting out carb snacks and switching to blackberries helped me lose weight and get in shape.

But, folks, let me say this: Man cannot live snacking on blackberries alone. Especially when he's having company, or when it's cocktail hour and it's time for something a little more substantial. I love to entertain my family and friends, but the bar is a little higher for me than for most people. Because I'm known for cooking the world's best barbecue, people who come to my house expect me to lay out a spread that's uniformly delicious. Does it frustrate me that my guests have high standards for me? Nope. In fact, I hate to disappoint them.

A lot of folks I meet are curious about what I eat when I'm at home. They ask me what I cook besides smoked meats, and by way of an answer this chapter is where I'd point them.

The simple answer is, I like all kinds of food, so long as it's good. When I decided to follow the Keto plan, I didn't want to give up my favorite snacks and appetizers. I realized that if I stuck to my usual routine of preparing simple dishes with good-quality ingredients and strong flavors, I could make snacks and apps in a Keto-style that would help me keep my weight down and my body healthy.

RECIPES

BBQ and Bacon Jalapeño Poppers with Ranch

MAKES 8 TO 10 POPPERS

The combination of a spicy pepper with a gooey, creamy filling is so addictive that it's made poppers very popular bar appetizers. A lot of folks don't realize how easy it is to make them at home, not to mention the fact they are entirely Keto-friendly.

INGREDIENTS

1 8-ounce package cream cheese, softened

2 tablespoons BBQ Beef Rub (*page 96*)

8 ounces bacon, cooked until crisp, then crumbled

2 scallions, white and light green parts only, chopped

1½ cups shredded cheddar cheese

8 to 10 medium jalapeño peppers

Pitmaster's Buttermilk Ranch Dressing (*page 164*), or use a favorite sugar-free brand

1. Preheat oven to 350°F.

2. Coat a medium baking sheet with cooking spray and set aside.

3. In a medium bowl, combine the softened cream cheese, BBQ Rub, bacon, scallions, and ¾ cup of the shredded cheese.

4. Fill the cavity of each jalapeño half with the mixture, then top each with a little of the remaining shredded cheese and transfer it to the prepared baking sheet. Repeat with the remaining jalapeños and filling mixture.

5. Bake the poppers for 30 minutes, or until the tops turn golden brown and the cheese mixture bubbles.

6. Serve warm alongside Pitmaster Ranch Dressing for dipping.

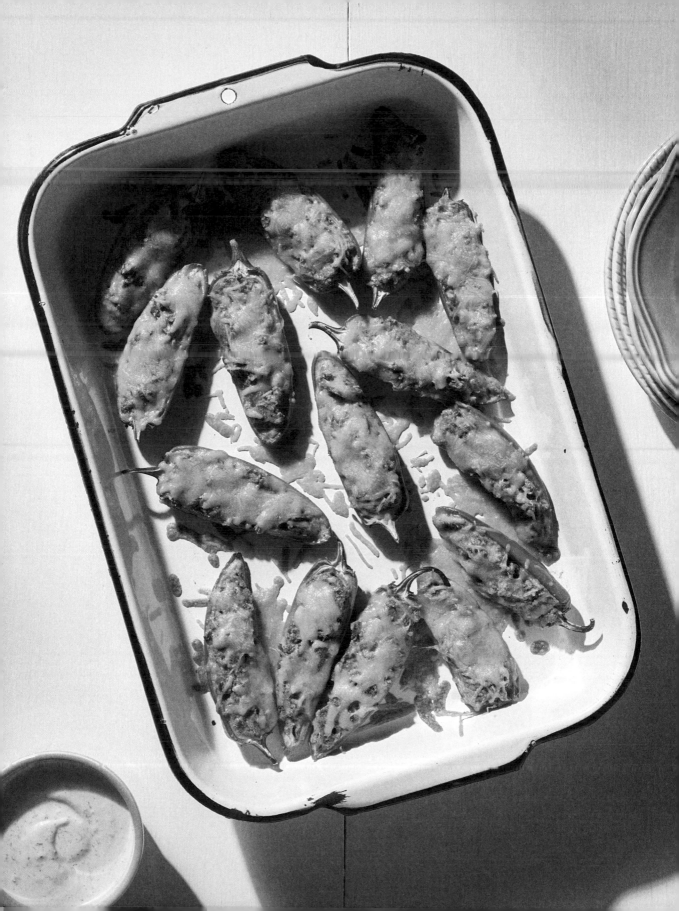

Classic Southern Deviled Eggs

MAKES 24 DEVILED EGGS

You might as well not have a picnic or a barbecue or any other friendly get-together in the state of Georgia If you're not planning to serve deviled eggs. This is one of our top comfort foods and they are naturally Keto. The following recipe is a basic traditional formula for textbook deviled eggs. On the occasions when I have some leftover smoked meat, I might throw some of it into the filling, too. And you can always gussy these up with the addition of pickle relish or crumbled bacon, both of which are excellent additions.

INGREDIENTS

12 large eggs

½ cup mayonnaise

¼ cup full-fat sour cream

1 tablespoon ground mustard

Kosher salt

1 tablespoon BBQ Beef Rub (*page 96*)

1. Hard boil the eggs: Gently place the eggs in a large saucepan and cover with about 3 inches of water. Bring the water to a boil, turn off the heat, cover the pot, and let sit for 20 minutes. Gently drain the eggs and fill the pan with cold water. Let sit for five minutes. One by one, lightly tap the eggs on the countertop to crack them open. Under a light stream of cold running water, take care to gently peel the eggs without damaging them. Pat each dry and let rest on paper towels while you unpeel the rest.

2. Use a clean sharp paring knife to halve the eggs lengthwise, wiping down the knife after each egg. Use a small spoon to carefully remove the yolks and transfer them to a small bowl. When all the yolks are removed, use a fork to mash them. Add the mayonnaise, sour cream, mustard, salt, and rub. Mix until smooth, tasting for seasoning and adjusting as you like.

3. Use a small spoon to fill the egg white "cups" with the yolk mixture; if you have a cake-decorating piping bag, you can use that, too. Sprinkle the eggs with a little more rub on top of each and refrigerate, covered loosely with plastic wrap, until ready to serve.

BBQ Keto Cocktail Meatballs

MAKES 4 SNACK SERVINGS

Cocktail meatballs are a fun throwback to that Frank Sinatra Rat Pack era. They're great pass-around appetizers. I like mine saucy and sticky, but not sweet—that's not how we do it on Keto. These are smoky, salty, and tangy. Eat 'em while you're playing "My Way" on your stereo.

INGREDIENTS

1 pound ground beef

½ cup plus two tablespoons grated Parmesan cheese

¼ cup homemade (or store-bought) pork rinds, crushed

1 teaspoon BBQ Beef Rub (*page 96*)

2 cloves minced garlic

1 large egg

1 tablespoon butter

2 teaspoons olive oil

Kosher salt and pepper

½ cup Tangy Sweet BBQ Sauce (*page 32*) or another sugar-free BBQ sauce

1. In a large bowl gently stir to combine the beef, parm, crushed pork rinds, rub, garlic, and egg. Season with salt and pepper and then shape into 1-inch balls.

2. In a large skillet over medium-high heat, melt the butter but do not allow it to brown. Add the olive oil. Add the meatballs and sear them on all sides until browned. Reduce the heat and add the sauce. Gently simmer, covered, for 10 minutes.

3. Skewer each meatball with a toothpick, arrange on platter, and enjoy with your libation of choice.

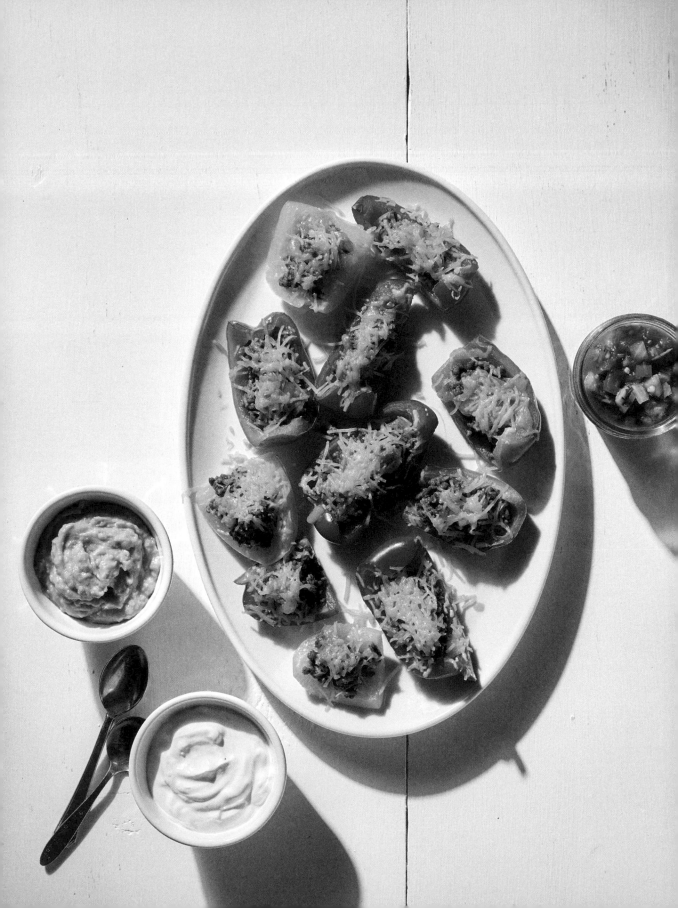

Keto BBQ Nachos

SERVES 2 TO 4

Y'all already know that I don't care for "fake" versions of real foods. These nachos are not made with tortilla chips, but that doesn't mean they don't deliver the same satisfaction as your favorite taco joint's version. What's great about making nachos on bell peppers is the fact that the pepper sections can hold up the toppings and add extra flavor to the everyone's favorite appetizer.

INGREDIENTS

2 medium bell peppers, a mix of red, yellow, and green

1 tablespoon vegetable oil

¼ teaspoon chili powder

½ teaspoon ground cumin

4 ounces ground beef

Kosher salt and freshly grated black pepper

1 cup shredded sharp cheddar cheese

½ cup chopped avocado

¼ cup pico de gallo

2 tablespoons full-fat sour cream

1. Line a medium baking sheet with foil.

2. Cut each bell pepper into sixths, then carefully remove the stem and seeds from each section taking care not to rip the peppers. Transfer the peppers to a medium microwave-safe bowl, add a tablespoon of water to the bowl, then cover it tightly with plastic wrap. Microwave the peppers on high until they are softened and pliable, about 3½ to 4 minutes. Let the pepper slices cool slightly, then arrange them cut-side up and close together on the prepared baking sheet and set aside.

3. In a large nonstick skillet over medium-high heat, warm the oil. Add the chili powder and cumin. Cook, stirring together, until fragrant and combined, about 30 seconds. Add the ground beef and cook, stirring and breaking into pieces, until browned and cooked through, about 4 minutes. Season to taste with salt and pepper and set aside.

4. Preheat the broiler.

5. Spoon some beef mixture onto each pepper piece. Sprinkle the cheese all over the beef and peppers. Broil until the cheese melts, about 30 seconds.

6. Remove the nachos from the broiler and top with dollops of avocado, pico de gallo, and sour cream. Serve immediately.

Pitmaster Pimento Cheese Spread

MAKES ABOUT 1½ CUPS

Everybody knows that pimento cheese spread is as Southern as Southern can be—it's our region's most important . . . well, what is it? It's a spread, it's a dip, it's a condiment, and no family picnic or barbecue would be the same without it. The good news is, it's naturally a Keto-friendly thing to eat; there are no carbs and no sugar in my pimento cheese recipe. Just make sure you don't spread it on crackers or toast—use a celery stalk or a carrot stick or a pork rind instead. This is also delicious spread on a burger, too.

INGREDIENTS

8 ounces extra-sharp cheddar cheese

¼ cup softened cream cheese

½ cup jarred pimento or other roasted red peppers, diced

¼ cup mayonnaise

½ teaspoon chile pepper flakes

1. In a large bowl, combine all the ingredients and gently stir with a rubber spatula or wooden spoon to combine until the mixture is smooth, about 1 minute. Cover tightly and store in the refrigerator until ready to use. Pimento cheese can be stored in the fridge for a week.

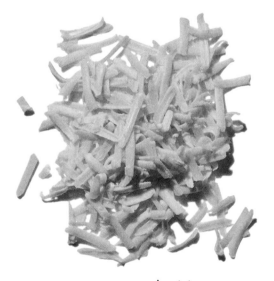

cheddar cheese

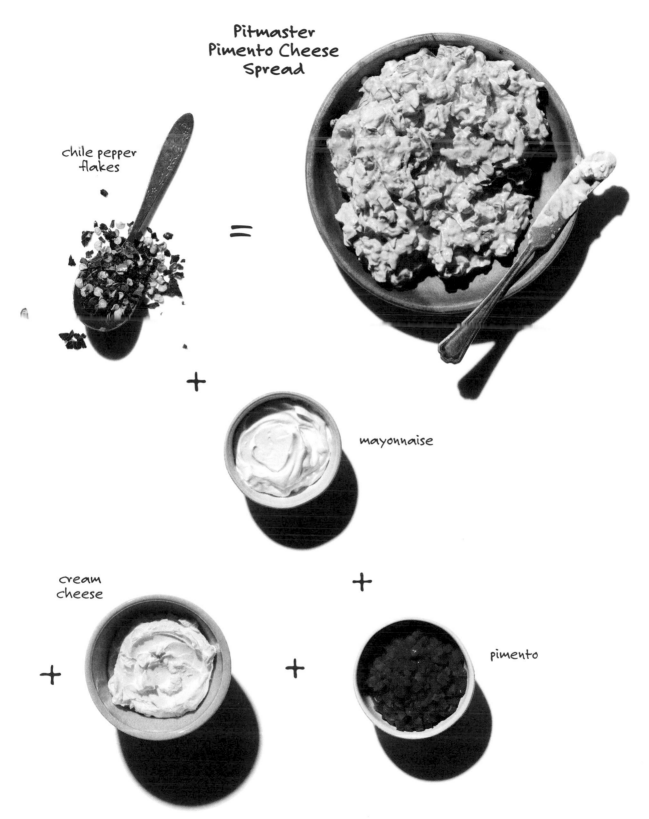

Pitmaster
Pimento Cheese
Spread

chile pepper
flakes

=

+

mayonnaise

cream
cheese

+

+

pimento

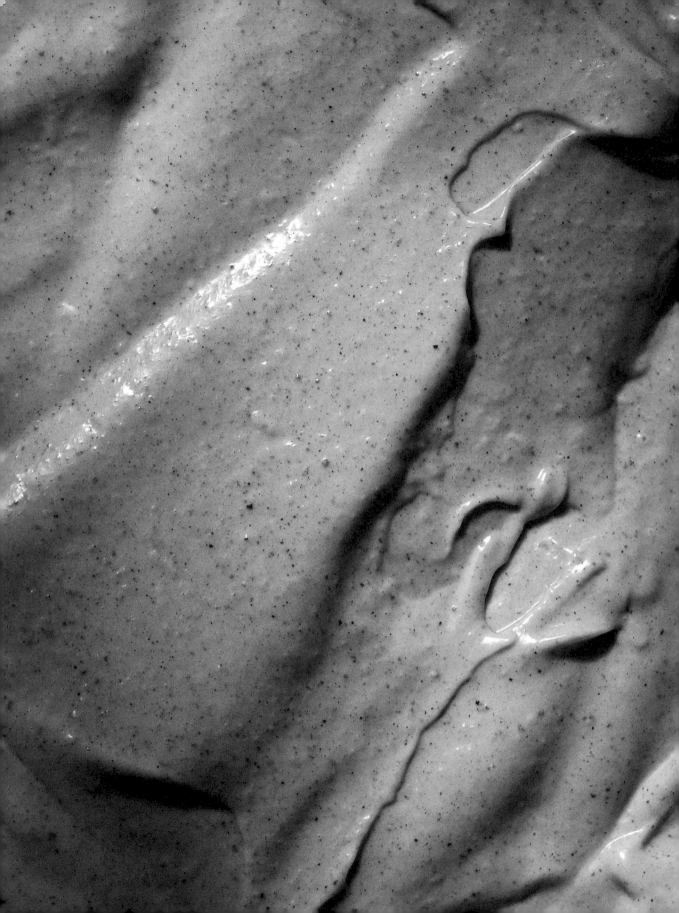

CHAPTER 7

Condiments

CONDIMENTS ARE ESSENTIAL for the "strong flavor" bit I've mentioned throughout this book. They are essential for a BBQ Keto follower. We eat a lot of foods like smoked meats and vegetables that benefit from the kind of flavor enhancers that condiments provide. I was delighted to discover that I could eat as much ranch dressing, blue cheese dressing, and spicy mayo as I wanted on my new so-called diet. Didn't make it feel too hard. And you're going to agree.

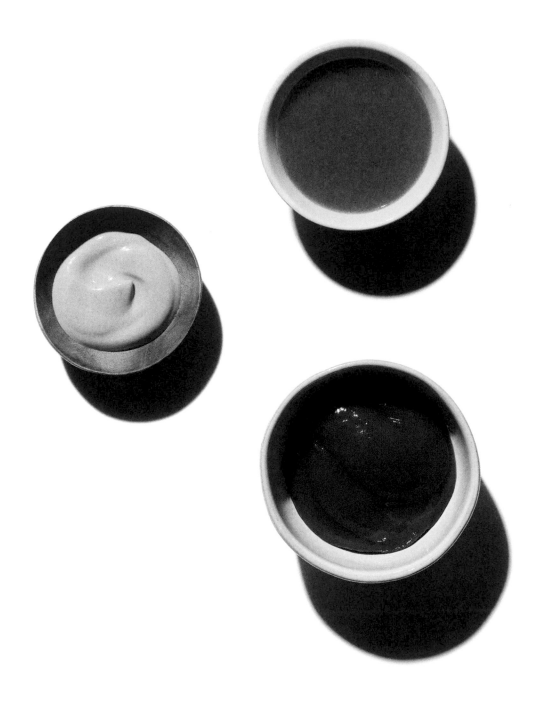

RECIPES

Keto "Honey" Mustard Sauce

I love honey mustard dressing and would pour some on just about anything. You can use this recipe as a salad dressing, a marinade, a sauce over cooked meat, or a condiment. Instead of honey, I use my favorite non-sugar sweetener, monk fruit sweetener, to soften these bold flavors.

INGREDIENTS

¼ cup cider vinegar

¼ cup olive oil

2 tablespoons mayonnaise

1 tablespoon spicy mustard

¼ cup yellow mustard

2 cloves garlic, minced

1 teaspoon Worcestershire sauce

1 tablespoon monk fruit sweetener (*see page 19*)

Kosher salt and freshly grated black pepper

1. In a medium bowl, whisk together all ingredients to combine. You can use an immersion blender to do this if you have one, but it's not required. Taste and adjust seasonings. Cover and store in the refrigerator until ready to use. This dressing can be refrigerated in a jar or another container with a lid and stored for a month.

Pitmaster's Buttermilk Ranch Dressing

MAKES ABOUT 1½ CUPS

You do not need me to tell you that you can use ranch as a dipping sauce for fresh vegetables, or a marinade for grilled chicken or pork, or a side dipping sauce for . . . just about anything you put in your mouth. I add a little smoky flavor to my version, and I like a ranch that has a lot of herbs plus the tang of buttermilk.

INGREDIENTS

1 cup buttermilk

½ cup full-fat sour cream

¼ cup mayonnaise

1 tablespoon vegetable oil

2 tablespoons cider vinegar

1 tablespoon dried parsley

1 teaspoon dried oregano

1 teaspoon dried dill

1 teaspoon BBQ Beef Rub (*page 96*) or your favorite sugar-free barbecue rub

1 teaspoon kosher salt

1. In a medium bowl, whisk together all ingredients to combine. Taste and adjust seasonings. Cover and store in the refrigerator until ready to use. This dressing can be refrigerated in a jar or other container with a lid and stored for up to five days.

Blue Cheese Dressing

MAKES ABOUT 2 CUPS

When I first tried the Keto lifestyle, I noticed that condiments were an important way to give my food more flavor. I was happy about that, because I love blue cheese dressing (see my Pitmaster Iceberg Wedge Salad with Bacon, page 134). The key to mine is equal parts blue cheese and mayonnaise, which I believe gives this dressing the perfect consistency.

INGREDIENTS

1 cup crumbled blue cheese

⅔ cup full-fat sour cream

⅔ cup mayonnaise

¼ cup fresh lemon juice

1 teaspoon garlic powder

Kosher salt and freshly ground black pepper

OPTIONAL: 2 scallions, white and light green parts only, minced, ½ teaspoon lemon zest

1. In a medium bowl, whisk together all ingredients to combine. Taste and adjust seasonings. Cover and store in the refrigerator until ready to use. This dressing can be refrigerated in a jar or other container with a lid and stored for up to five days.

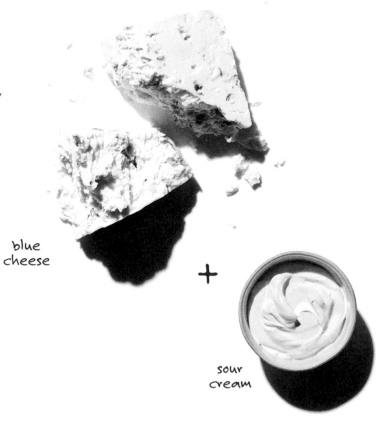

blue cheese

+

sour cream

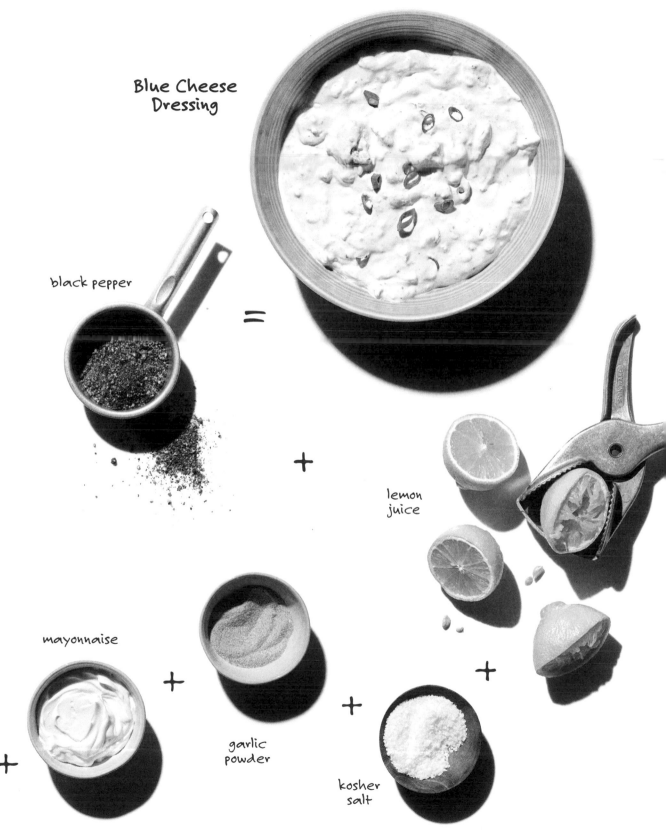

Blue Cheese
Dressing

black pepper

=

+

lemon
juice

mayonnaise

+

garlic
powder

+

kosher
salt

+

+

Green Goddess Dressing

I never knew it until recently—probably because like many folks I was introduced to Green Goddess dressing in my supermarket grocery store aisle—but this was invented in the 1920s in San Francisco and is considered a California classic. Green Goddess needs to have a lot of green herbs in it to give it bite and punch; here's my formula, but you can feel free to add any chopped green herbs or spices you like to yours. Fresh chopped parsley and chives are delicious additions if you have some around.

INGREDIENTS

¼ cup buttermilk

¼ cup full-fat sour cream

1 teaspoon cider vinegar or fresh lemon juice

1 garlic clove, minced

1 tablespoon olive oil

1 teaspoon dried oregano

1 teaspoon dried tarragon

1. In a medium bowl, whisk together all ingredients to combine. Taste and adjust seasonings. Cover and store in the refrigerator until ready to use. This dressing can be refrigerated in a jar or other container with a lid and stored for up to five days.

Spicy Mayo

MAKES ABOUT 1 CUP

This dressing is damn near unbeatable if you spread it on a burger, then wrap that burger up in some crisp, cold iceberg lettuce leaves. Delicious.

INGREDIENTS

1 cup mayonnaise

¼ cup sriracha sauce

2 teaspoons BBQ Beef Rub (*page 96*)

Dash or two of hot sauce

1. In a small bowl whisk together all of the ingredients until well combined. Cover and store in the refrigerator until ready to use. This dressing can be refrigerated in a jar or other container with a lid and stored for up to five days.

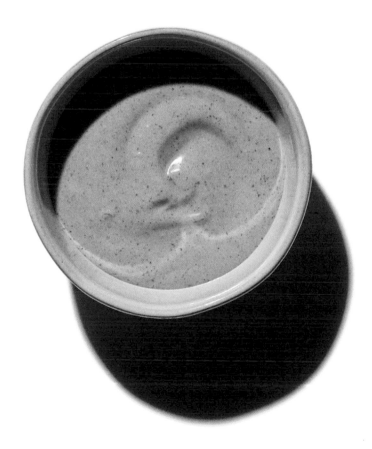

Garlic Green Mayo

When I started researching the Keto diet, I noticed right away that mayonnaise seemed to be the top condiment for Keto followers. This is because as long as you don't add sugar to it, it has no carbs. When I was on the diet for a while, I started looking for ways to make my mayo a little more interesting and flavorful, and this is one of my best concoctions.

INGREDIENTS

1 cup mayonnaise

4 large garlic cloves, minced

Juice of 1 lemon

1 teaspoon dried parsley

1 teaspoon dried oregano

OPTIONAL: 1 teaspoon chives, whites and light green parts only, chopped

1. In a small bowl whisk together all of the ingredients until well combined. Cover and store in the refrigerator until ready to use. This dressing can be refrigerated in a jar or other container with a lid and stored for up to five days.

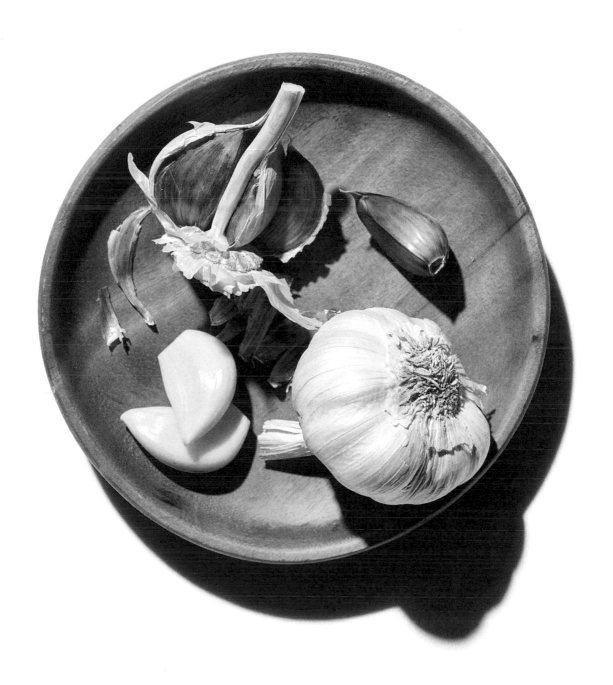

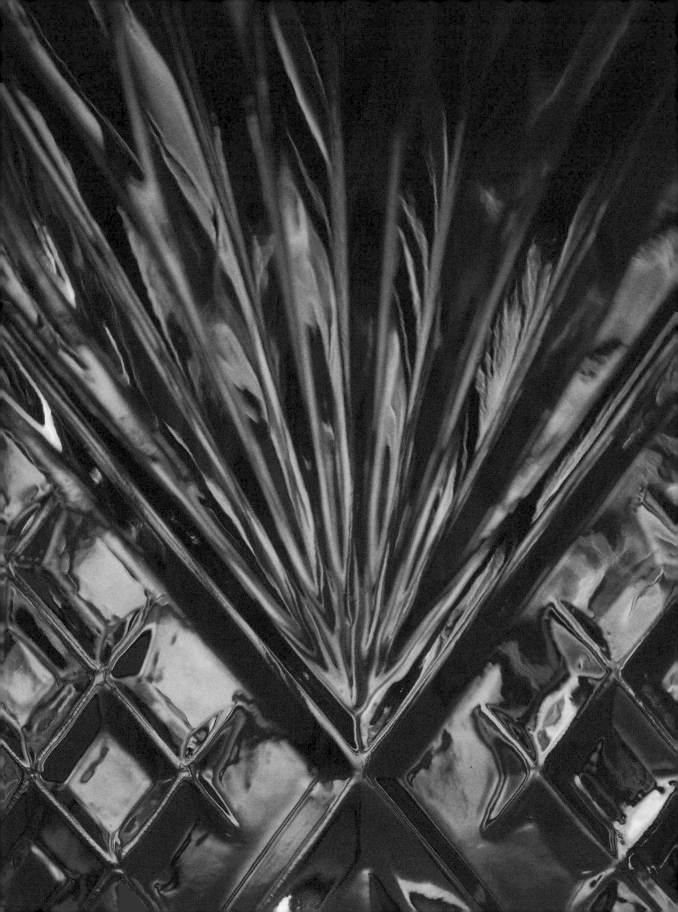

CHAPTER 8

Drinks

JUST BECAUSE YOU'VE GOT A KETO PLAN TO FOLLOW DOESN'T MEAN YOU CAN'T HAVE A LITTLE FUN. Part of the reason I chose the Keto plan when I was good and ready to drop some pounds and improve my health is because drinking alcohol on Keto is just fine, so long as you know what to drink and you keep it in moderation.

That's right: There are plenty of low-carb drinks you can have that allow your body to maintain a state of ketosis (What's ketosis, again? See page 17). Why? Because hard liquor itself has no carbs and will not kick you out of ketosis. Alcohol is not sugar and does not spike blood sugar, which is what kicks you out of ketosis. What you might mix it with, however, is a different story. Here's my guide:

KETO YES:

HARD LIQUOR: Vodka, rum, tequila, gin, brandy, whiskey, etc. Most of these have zero carbs.

LIGHT BEER: Most light beers are fine, but check the carb counts of your favorite brands.

HARD SELTZERS: These are basically seltzer waters spiked with a flavor. Make sure you buy the brands that have no sugar added.

DRY MARTINI: Made with either vodka or gin, you can have it shaken or stirred, with a twist or dirty with olives. Just make sure there's no added fruit juice or sweet liqueurs.

VODKA AND SODA: . . . or gin and soda, tequila and soda, whiskey and soda. As long as you remember to mix your booze with club soda and not with tonic, which contains added sugar, you're good. A wedge of lemon or lime is your best friend in this department.

DRY RED OR DRY WHITE WINE: While wine is not completely carb-free, a dry red like a Cabernet Sauvignon or a dry white like a Pinot Noir only contains a couple carbs, so you can plan your day accordingly. Note: The same is not true for dessert wines like port or sherry, or sweet wines like Riesling. Forget you even heard of those.

KETO NO:

MOST MIXED DRINKS: Avoid anything with simple syrup (sugar syrup), agave, margarita mix, sweet and sour mix, and anything mixed with sugary soda, such as Coca-Cola or ginger ale, or juice, any sweet wines, hard ciders, or wine coolers.

See there? You have more "yes" than "no" items. And you have the following recipes for my favorite cocktails on the planet. Of course, on some days nothing beats a good glass of your favorite liquor, served neat, no mixer required.

How about non-alcoholic drinks?

KETO YES:

Nearly anything without **SUGAR**, like flavored waters.

KETO NO:

Put down the **SWEET TEA**. It's got way too much sugar. Skip most **SODAS**. Even the sugar-free ones. **FRUIT JUICES**, like orange juice, are packed with sugar and thus carbs. **DAIRY MILK**.

RECIPES

The Skinny Pitmaster Mint-Basil 'Rita

I noticed a few years back that "skinny" cocktails were all the rage. Well, I'm no trend follower, but I am skinnier now. Here's my version of a skinny margarita, enhanced by combining mint and basil, two of my favorite herbs. It's a little different from the usual formula, but trust me, it'll have the same results.

INGREDIENTS

6 tablespoons fresh lime juice

8 leaves fresh mint

8 leaves fresh basil

2 cups ice cubes

3 ounces (6 tablespoons) tequila or rum

1 cup sparkling water

1. In a medium bowl, combine the lime juice with the mint and basil leaves. Use a muddler or other tool to muddle the leaves and fruit, crushing them in the lime juice as best as possible. Divide the muddled juice and herbs between two standard margarita glasses.

2. Fill the glasses ¾ of the way with ice. Add 1½ ounces (3 tablespoons) of tequila or rum to each glass. Fill the glasses to the top with the sparkling water. Gently stir the cocktail with a stirrer or a long, thin spoon.

Pitmaster's Bloody Mary

MAKES 2 COCKTAILS

To hell with brunch, this drink right here is almost a meal in itself. Sometimes I like a Bloody Mary with tequila instead of the traditional vodka, but you're welcome to use the spirit of choice.

INGREDIENTS

2 teaspoons smoked paprika

2 teaspoons celery salt

2 cups ice

2 ounces (¼ cup) vodka or tequila

6 ounces (¾ cups) tomato juice

Juice of 1 lemon

Few dashes hot sauce

½ cup BBQ Keto Strong Beef Broth (*page 100*)

OPTIONAL: fresh dill pickle spear, lemon wedge, 1 thick-cut piece of grilled steak

1. Get two 16-ounce mason jars, mugs, or highball cocktail glasses. On a small plate or in a shallow bowl, combine the smoked paprika and celery salt and stir to combine. Moisten the rim of your cocktail glass of choice with a little water, and then turn the rim around in the mixture a few times to coat it to your liking. Repeat with second glass.

2. Fill your glasses with ice. Add the remaining ingredients to your glasses of ice one at a time in the order given. Give the drinks a good stir. I like to use a long handled iced tea spoon, but use any spoon that'll fit into your glass.

3. Garnish the drinks as you like and serve. I put in a pickle, lemon wedge, and even a piece of steak.

The Cowboy

MAKES 1 COCKTAIL

It's spicy, it's rustic, it will put hair on your chest, and make you feel like you're ready to ride your horse into the sunset. If you prefer a less spicy version, skip the serrano pepper. (If you want to stay fully Keto BBQ, you need to know that monk fruit sweetener can be hard to dissolve in liquid. So give your drink some extra shakes and stirs to get the job done, that's what I do.)

INGREDIENTS

4 ounces (½ cup) whiskey or tequila, preferably reposado tequila (like Cabo Wabo® Reposado Tequila)

Juice of 1 lime

8 ounces (1 cup) unsweetened iced tea (*page 179*)

1 teaspoon monk fruit sweetener, depending on desired sweetness (*see page 19*)

1 serrano pepper, cut in half vertically

2 lime wedges, for garnish

1. Fill two 16-ounce mason jars, mugs, or highball cocktail glasses with ice. Add equal amounts of whiskey or tequila to each glass, then equal amounts of lime juice, iced tea, and monk fruit sweetener to each glass.

2. Give each drink a good stir; I like to use a long-handled iced tea spoon but any spoon that'll fit into your glass will do. Give a few extra stirs to dissolve the monk fruit sweetener.

3. Add half a serrano pepper to each glass and a lime wedge. Now go ride 'em, cowboy.

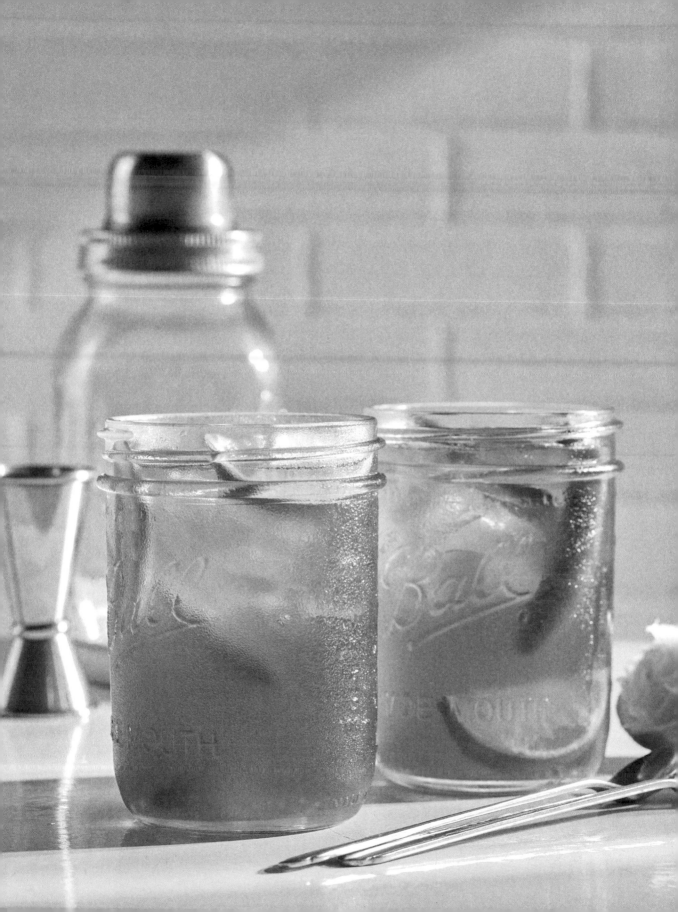

The Keto-jito

This is my version of a mojito. Even though monk fruit sweetener is my all-purpose Keto-approved sweetener of choice, it's a bit harder to dissolve it. You can use a packet of Splenda or Stevia here if you prefer and it will be a bit easier. But I think having to give the monk fruit sweetener a few extra stirs is worth it.

INGREDIENTS

2 limes, each cut into 4 wedges

About 16 fresh mint leaves

4 ounces (½ cup) white rum

2 cups ice cubes

½ to 1 teaspoon monk fruit sweetener, depending on desired sweetness (*see page 19*)

Sparkling water

1. Divide the lime wedges and mint leaves between two tall highball-style cocktail glasses. Reserve 2 or 3 mint leaves for garnish. Use a muddler or other tool (such as the bottom of a wooden spoon) to crush the leaves and lime quarters and release their juices and oils.

2. Divide the rum, ice, and monk fruit sweetener evenly between the glasses. Give the drink a good stir; I like to use a long handled iced tea spoon but any spoon that'll fit in the glass will work. Give a few extra stirs to dissolve the monk fruit sweetener. Top off with sparkling water. Serve garnished with a mint leaf.

Keto Iced Tea

You can make this basic formula for unsweetened iced tea with any kind of tea you like. I like peach tea the best, but I know plenty of folks out there like green tea. You can add any flavorings you get a hankering for—orange and peach slices are great. The key is replacing the huge amounts of sugar that are in sweet tea with fruit and other flavors. Also, come cocktail hour, you can always spike this tea with a shot of whatever you like. Bourbon and vodka are ideal choices.

INGREDIENTS

2 tea bags of your choice

Flavorings, such as lemon slices, orange slices, and fresh mint leaves

4 cups cold water

2 cups ice cubes

1. In a pitcher, combine the tea bags, flavorings, and 2 cups of the cold water. Refrigerate for at least 1 hour and as long as 2 hours.

2. After 2 hours, remove the tea bags and either discard the flavorings or replace them with fresh ones, depending on your taste and preferences. Add the remaining cold water. Serve poured over ice.

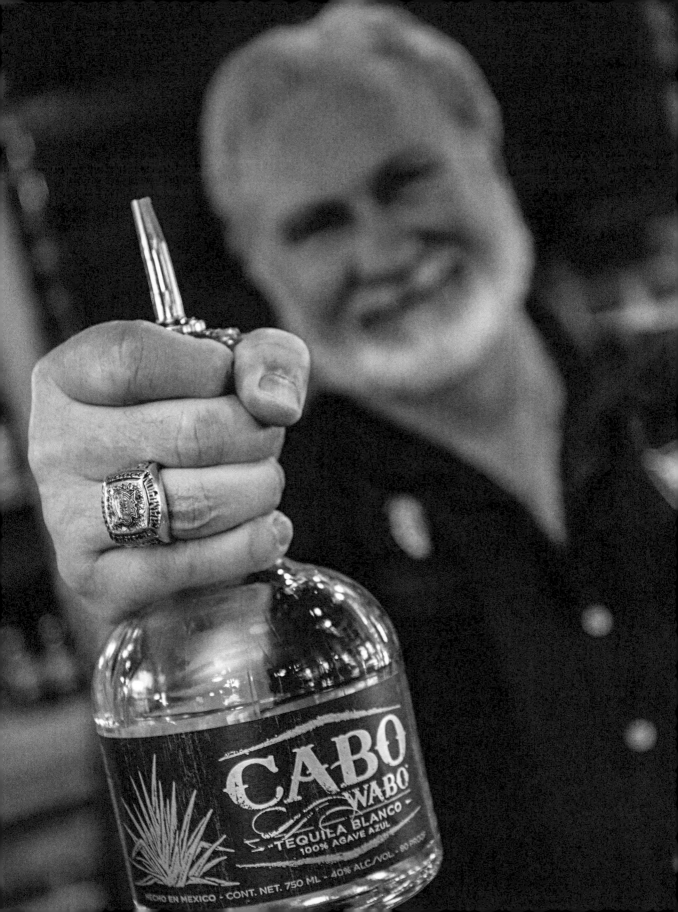

Spicy Strawberry 'Rita

MAKES 2 COCKTAILS

I defy you to find a more refreshing drink on a hot summer night than this cocktail. The fresher the strawberries the sweeter it will be, but frozen strawberries are a perfect substitute. If you don't care for spicy cocktails, skip coating the rims of the glasses.

INGREDIENTS

2 teaspoons kosher salt

2 teaspoons mild, medium or hot chili powder

6 fresh strawberries, hulled

2 ounces (¼ cup) light rum or tequila, preferably blanco tequila (like Cabo Wabo® Blanco Tequila)

Juice of 1 lime, freshly squeezed

1 tablespoon water

4 large ice cubes

½ teaspoon monk fruit sweetener, optional (*see page 19*)

1 lime wedge, optional garnish

1. Combine the salt and chili powder on a plate or in a shallow bowl. Moisten the rim of two 16-ounce mason jars, mugs, or highball cocktail glasses with a little water. Turn the rim of each glass in the mixture a few times to coat it to your liking.

2. In the container of a blender, pulse the strawberries, rum or tequila, lime juice, water, and ice cubes. Blend the mixture until smooth.

3. Taste for sweetness. Depending on the strawberries and your personal taste, you might find that it is sweet enough for you. If not, add ½ teaspoon of monk fruit sweetener to the blender and blend again for 30 seconds. If it's still not sweet enough for you, add a little more.

4. If you prefer to remove the strawberry seeds, strain the mixture through a fine mesh sieve into your prepared glasses. If you don't care about those little seeds, as I don't, just pour it right in and start drinking.

Refreshing Flavored Water

Flavored water is something that has gotten me through the Keto diet and helped keep me in ketosis. As boring as it may sound, drinking lots of water keeps you hydrated, helps stave off cravings for sweets, and is a healthy habit to get into. Because it's so easy to flavor water, I'm not going to give you a recipe for it, just this method:

Fill a large pitcher with water. Add the flavorings of your choice including fresh raspberries, fresh mint leaves, grapefruit slices, or cucumber slices. Just a small handful or a few slices is enough to flavor an entire pitcher of water. Let it sit in the refrigerator for at least 1 hour or as long as 2 hours. After 2 hours, remove the flavorings. That's it. It's that easy to make drinking enough water every day a little bit more interesting for you.

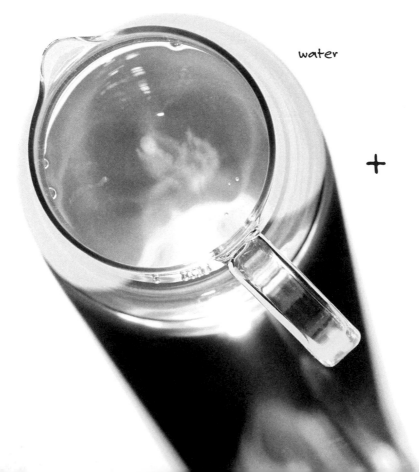

water

+

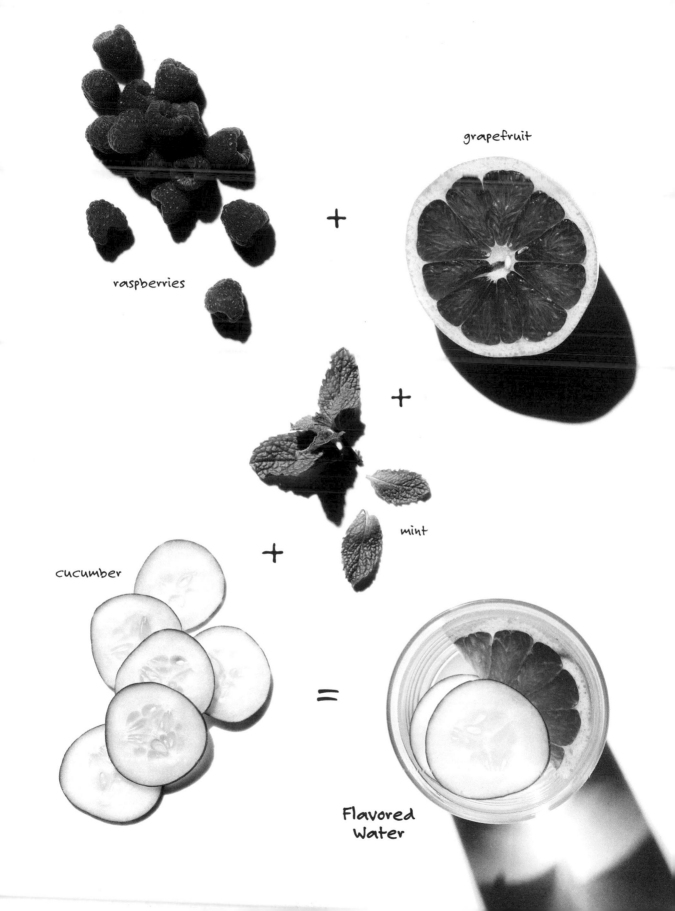

raspberries

grapefruit

+

+

mint

cucumber

+

=

Flavored Water

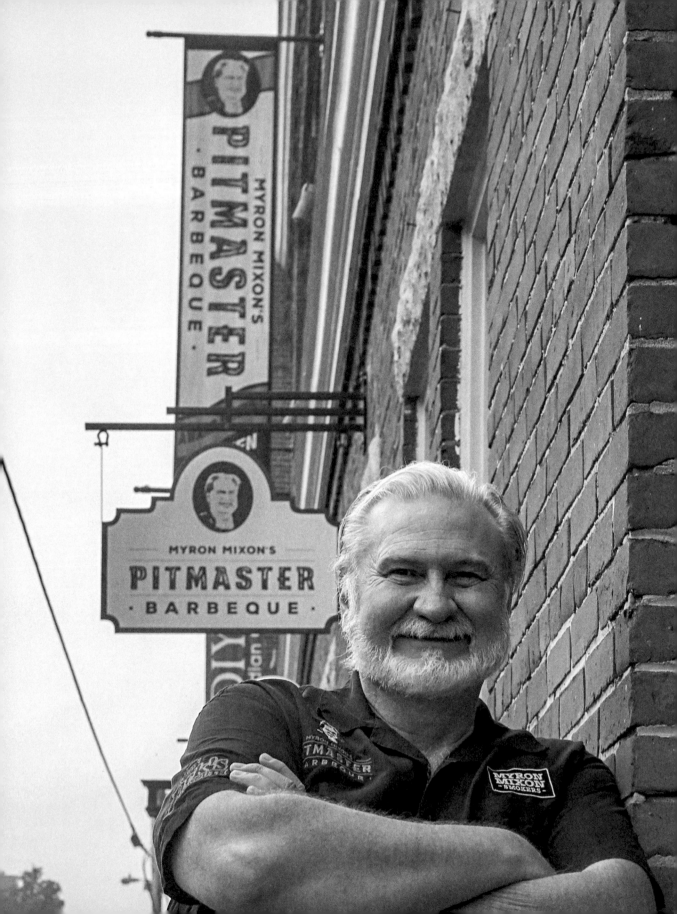

A NOTE ABOUT
RESTAURANTS
& EXERCISE

LOOK, I CANNOT TELL YOU THAT IT'S EASY TO LOSE MORE THAN 100 POUNDS. I would be lying. But I can tell you that I have done it and that it was worth it. I've already given the recipes I've used to change the way I eat, but also have to discuss two other big things that helped me to take off the weight and keep it off.

Once I figured out how the Keto diet worked and how to manage my meals, which is what all those recipes that I just gave you are for, the two things I had left to figure out were:

1. What to do in restaurants so I could still go out to eat with family and friends and enjoy myself?

2. How to work in an exercise plan that wasn't so regimented that it was going to drive me crazy?

Here is the short and sweet cheat sheet for how I solved those two problems.

Restaurants

When I made up my mind to lose weight, I went to the bookstore. I'm old-fashioned like that: I like flipping through books I can hold in my hands, and I don't always want to use my tablet when I want to read something. I noticed that almost all the diet books I looked at start out with all the things you can't do; most of them say *you can't eat this,* and *you can't eat that,* and, worst of all to me, because I love to go out to eat and pick up takeout when I'm not working, most diets tell you to *avoid restaurants.* Now, if you don't make a diet plan one that lets people live the way they want to and still follow it, it's going be too rigid. Sooner or later, people will fall back on doing the things they like to do and recycle that book. Keto is a good choice for folks because you don't have to give up anything you really love—unless maybe you own a donut shop. In that case you might be screwed. For me and the rest of us, I can tell you that there's always something I can find to eat on any restaurant menu in the world that will allow me to stay on Keto. If you like meat and you like some vegetables, you'll be just fine on the Keto plan. Most diets tell you to avoid restaurants in the first place because they want you to cut down on fat, in particular high-fat, high-calorie ingredients like butter, cream, and cheese. But Keto wants you to train your body to burn fat instead of carbs, which means that loading up on those foods is just fine. All of those no-no ingredients on other diets that are so prevalent in restaurant cooking—your butter, cream, and cheese—you can have 'em.

I have just two rules I follow whenever I know I'm going to a restaurant, ordering in food, or picking up takeout:

A. First, remind yourself what a carb is. A carb is a starch or a sugar. Complex carbs are starches like potatoes, grains, and beans. Simple starches are sugars and sweeteners like white sugar and also honey, maple syrup, and brown sugar. Recall what I already told you: Some fruits and vegetables are higher in carbs than others (*see my list of the ones to avoid for that reason on page 21*). Also recall the fact that no meats contain carbs unless some have been added in their preparation, usually in sauces or as side dishes, so as long as you order a grilled piece of meat, fowl, or fish, you're all set.

B. Don't order anything with lots of carbs—like bread, rice, or pasta.

Believe it or not, those two rules leave us with plenty of options. This is true even at steakhouses. I like steakhouses, but only visit them once a month or so as a treat to myself because I try to watch my red meat intake to stay heart-healthy. Here's what I get when I go: an iceberg wedge and a ribeye. I don't need anything else. At other places, I still order sandwiches and burgers and peel them back so that I eat what's inside but not the buns. Guess what? It does not bother me. I'm perfectly happy to have double meat and veggies on a sandwich and skip the bun. I still get full, only I'm not filling up on bread.

When I go to a restaurant, I often look at the creamy soups and try those—I can have all the lobster bisque I want and still lose weight. I can have all the cheese I want. I can have grilled chicken and fish, as much as I want. I just make sure that I substitute all the starchy sides like mashed potatoes with double veggies or a side salad instead. At Mexican restaurants, I order fajitas and fill my plate with the meat, grilled vegetables, guacamole, and sour cream—I do not need the tortillas. At Chinese restaurants, I skip the rice. My favorite dessert is blackberries with heavy cream poured over them—just about any restaurant worth its salt will make that for you even if it's not on the menu, and there ain't nothing better.

Exercise

As I write this today, I'm fifty-eight years old. I have had orthoscopic surgery on my knee. My job involves standing on my feet for hours and hours at a time. I'm not looking to get injured or put any additional pressure on this old body. That means I'm not going to the gym just to pick up a bunch of weights, and I'm not doing any stationary bike-pedaling that will send me right back to the orthopedic surgeon. I do not need some twenty-three-year-old fit-as-a-fiddle person yelling at me like a drill sergeant telling me to drop and give him twenty. I don't need someone in a matching workout outfit telling me I'm the best and that I can do anything I set my mind to.

However, I know that cardio is important to stay healthy. You have to get your heart rate up every day if you can, especially if you're trying to lose weight. But you get to pick how you want to do that. I have a big outdoor area on my property, but I don't love walking around in a damn circle. What I do like doing is waking up and getting on a treadmill for forty-five minutes every morning. I treat it like it's a job, like there aren't any questions about it that need to be asked, like I have to depend on it in order to survive. I like walking on my treadmill more than I like walking outside because I can make sure I'm going at a fast enough and at a steady enough clip to get my heartrate up. Walking on my treadmill every day, forty-five minutes a day, makes me healthy, and it keeps all the weight I've worked so hard to lose off me.

If all you do is walk for forty five minutes a day and pair that activity along with your Keto eating plan, I promise you that you will not only lose weight fast but will also keep it off. I'm not a motivational coach by any means, but I know how to set yourself up for success: Make a morning walk the first thing you do every day. You don't need to bother with weights, trainers, gadgets, or classes. I was so relieved to discover that I did not have to do three sets of any type of dumbbell curls. I do not miss doing squats, which I have always hated. Just like how I tell you that a Keto eating program has to have a plan you can follow that's easy enough to stick to or you'll drop off it, the same is true for exercising. The average human being just wants to get some weight off and make their life better, not become a bodybuilder. Don't beat yourself up. Don't subject yourself to some unnecessary body shaming. I know you can do this without a gym membership. The best advice I can give you: Get a damn treadmill for your house and get on it every day, no questions asked. That's how I did it.

If that's not what you're going to stick with, then you need to find what you will do every damn day. Don't make it something too hard or that you'll hate. Make it something that you can live with and you'll be thanking me later.

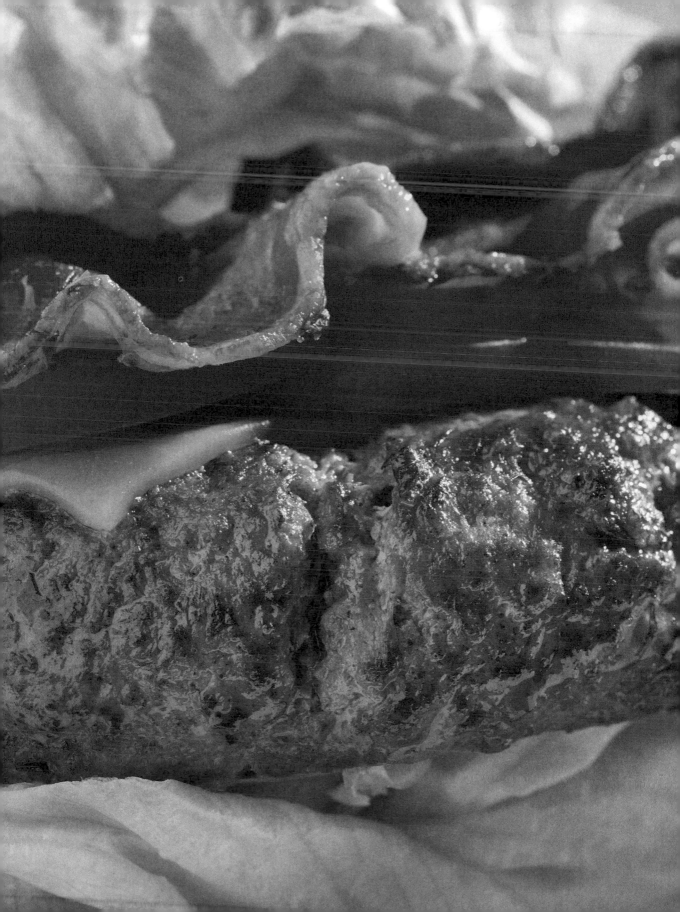

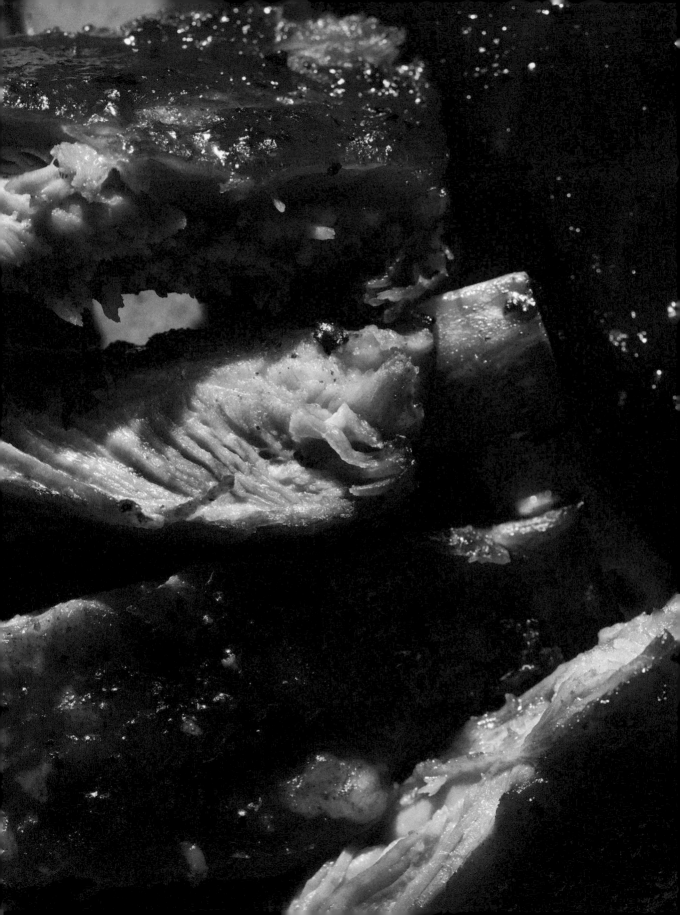

Myron Mixon

MYRON MIXON is a *New York Times* bestselling author of *Smokin' with Myron Mixon: Recipes Made Simple, from the Winningest Man in Barbecue* (May 2011), *Everyday Barbeque* (May 2013), *Myron Mixon's BBQ Rules* (2016), and *BBQ&A with Myron Mixon* (2019).

As a four-time world barbecue champion, Myron Mixon is the winningest man in barbecue. The chief cook of the Jack's Old South Competition Bar-B-Que Team, the mayor of Unadilla, Georgia, and chef/partner in Myron Mixon's Pitmaster BBQ with locations in Old Town Alexandria, Virginia; Miami, Florida; and Hoboken, New Jersey. (For more on Myron's restaurants, visit www.myronmixonbbq.com.)

Myron is the executive producer and host of *BBQ Rules,* host of *Smoked,* and star of *BBQ Pitmasters* and *BBQ Pit Wars* on Discovery's Destination America.

Myron has his own line of smokers, Myron Mixon Smokers (www.myronmixonsmokers.com), and a line of sauces, rubs, a three-in-one grill tool, rib skinner, and other barbecue products. He also runs a very successful BBQ cooking school in Unadilla, Georgia, and frequently does classes and cooking demos across the world. For more information on his products and classes, visit www.myronmixon.com.

Kelly Alexander
Writer

Kelly Alexander is a writer, editor, and anthropologist of food based in Chapel Hill, North Carolina. She has won a James Beard Journalism Award for her work on "forgotten food writer" Clementine Paddleford, and is the co-author of a *New York Times* bestselling cookbook on barbecue, *Smokin' with Myron Mixon*. She has written about food politics and culture for the *New York Times,* The *New Republic, Newsweek, O, The Oprah Magazine,* and many other publications. She holds a degree in journalism from Northwestern University's Medill School of Journalism and a Ph.D. in cultural anthropology from Duke University. When she's not working with Myron Mixon, she's a visiting professor of food studies at Duke's Center for Documentary Studies and in the American Studies Department at the University of North Carolina–Chapel Hill.

Rob DeBorde
Designer

Rob DeBorde is a writer and artist based in Portland, Oregon. His work has been featured in numerous cookbooks, magazines, restaurant menus, logos, neon signs, and other food-related enterprises. He is the author and illustrator of *Fish on a First-Name Basis,* an indispensable guide to all things wet and edible. Rob also wrote 50+ episodes of *Good Eats* and created the award-winning animated cooking show *Deep Fried, Live! with Tako the Octopus.* He moonlights as a writer of zombie westerns (*Portlandtown: A Tale of the Oregon Wyldes*) and magical video games (*Harry Potter: Magic Awakened*).   www.foragercreative.com

Dhanraj Emanuel
Photographer

Originally from India, Dhanraj Emanuel comes from a long line of photographers, including his father, uncle, and grandfather. He developed a passion for food after he moved to America and began to cook for himself. He brings together his love for cooking and photography by shooting all things food. For Dhanraj, food is essential—it's universal. It provides the ideal setting to connect and interact, to understand and celebrate each other. Food it seems is the common thread in our lives, sustenance for many, history, culture, and memory for some, but identity for all. His photographs seek to highlight the meaningful connections between people and food.   www.dhanrajemanuel.com

Dawn Longobardo
Food Stylist

Dawn Longobardo is a food stylist based in North Carolina. Her first memories circle around food. Her grandmother Rose was a master in the kitchen. Whether it was a holiday or just Tuesday pasta night, the family would linger at her giant kitchen table eating, talking, and laughing. Dawn fell in love with styling food as a young art director in NYC in 1986. Spending time with amazing photographers and stylists made her realize that she loved working in the studio as much as she did in that art department. That exposure prompted her to further her education at The Culinary Institute of America, where she graduated in 1996. She then moved to North Carolina and apprenticed with other stylists before going out on her own. She loves styling for print, video, publishing, and editorial. Dawn lives in Pittsboro with her husband, Ron, daughters Emily and Lila, and her sweet pup, Weeza.   www.dawnlongobardo.com

Michael Psaltis
Producer

Michael Psaltis runs the Culinary Entertainment Agency, a full-service literary and talent management firm specializing in the food world. He has represented chefs, writers and other talented individuals and brands for over two decades.   www.the-cea.com

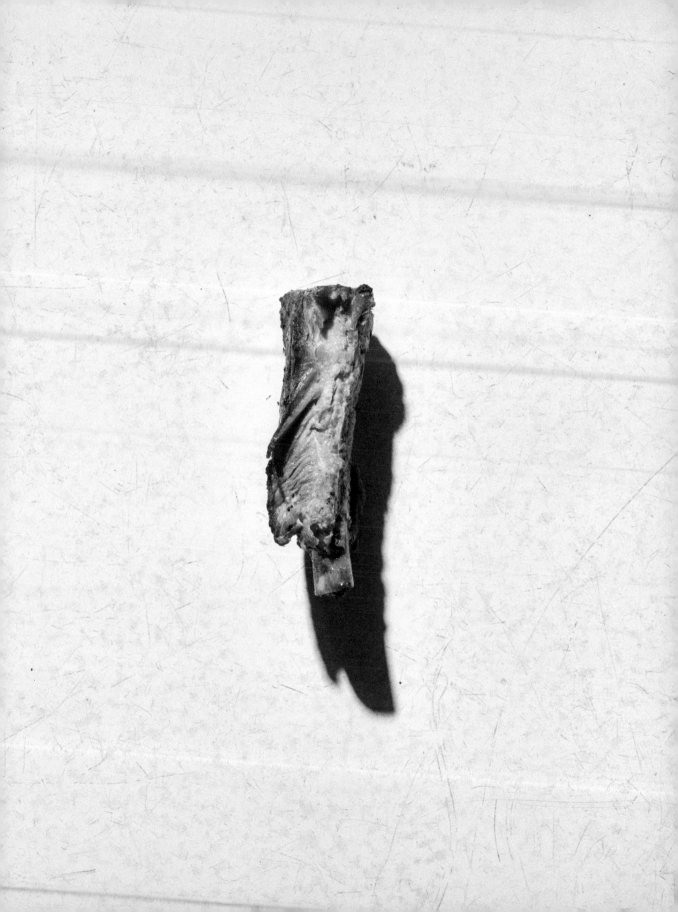

Editor: Garrett McGrath
Designer: Rob DeBorde
Production manager: Larry Pekarek

Library of Congress Control Number: 2020944097

ISBN: 978-1-4197-5118-9
eISBN: 978-1-64700-143-8

Printed and bound in the United States
10 9 8 7 6 5 4 3 2 1

Abrams books are available at special discounts when purchased in quantity for premiums and
promotions as well as fundraising or educational use. Special editions can also be created to specification.
For details, contact specialsales@abramsbooks.com or the address below.

Abrams® is a registered trademark of Harry N. Abrams, Inc.

ABRAMS The Art of Books
195 Broadway, New York, NY 10007
abramsbooks.com